BEING MENTALLY ILL

A SOCIOLOGICAL THEORY

Second Edition

BEING MENTALLY ILL

A SOCIOLOGICAL THEORY

Second Edition

Thomas J. Scheff

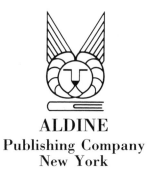

ALDINE
Publishing Company
New York

THE AUTHOR

Thomas J. Scheff, Professor of Sociology at the University of California, Santa Barbara, has been Associate Editor of the *American Sociological Review; Social Problems; Contemporary Sociology; The American Sociologist; Journal of Health and Social Behavior* and is Consulting Editor of the *American Journal of Sociology.* He is the author of Mental Illness and Social Processes; Labeling Madness; and Catharsis in Healing, Ritual and Drama.

First Edition published 1966
Aldine Publishing Company
200 Saw Mill River Road
Hawthorne, N.Y. 10532

Library of Congress Cataloging in Publication Data

Scheff, Thomas J.
  Being mentally ill.

  Includes index.
1   1. Mental illness—Social aspects. 2. Mental illness—
Etiology. 3. Social control. I. Title. [DNLM: 1. Social
desirability. 2. Mental disorders. WM 100 S316b]
RC454.4.S32   1984   362.2   84-6224
ISBN 0-202-30309-8
ISBN 0-202-30310-1 (pbk.)

Printed in the United States of America
10 9 8 7 6 5 4 3 2

Fernando Romero, chief of one of Mexico City's secret police corps, was attacked by a demented opponent in a hall near his office late Friday night. The attacker raised a razor against Romero when the latter opened the door to the hall. Romero immediately closed the door and called for his aides. The man was disarmed and brought to Romero who, realizing the man was insane, admonished him and sent him home.

México (D. F.) News

No point in cluttering up an asylum with a lot of nuts.

The New Yorker
May 15, 1965

We have endeavored . . . to observe a kind of perspective, that one part may cast light upon another.

Francis Bacon
Advancement of Learning

TABLE OF CONTENTS

IV REVIEW

PREFACE TO THE SECOND EDITION

THE first edition of this book was published in 1966. The research on which it was based was conducted during the period 1960–1964. Since that time, there have been many extraordinary changes in the field of mental illness: the introduction of tranquilizers on a massive scale in the treatment of mental illness; the discovery of the neurotransmitters; the proliferation and development of psychological therapies; the changes in the mental health laws governing commitment and treatment; and finally, the sizeable increase in the number and scope of social scientific studies of mental illness. This revision updates the earlier version and brings some of these changes and their aftereffects into its purview.

After due consideration, I decided to revise mainly by addition rather than by making large changes in the original text. Because I was unable to find a very concise statement of the theory of social control, I wrote a new chapter especially for this revision (Chapter 2) stating the main elements of the theory of social control and relating them to deviance and to mental illness. The remaining chapters that have been added are based on articles that I have published over the last sixteen years. Three studies (Chapters 7, 8, and 9) expand the section on research (Part II). Two new parts have been added: Part III, on controversies, and Part IV, which reviews and assesses the current status of the labeling theory of mental illness.

I have resisted the temptation to make large changes in the text that was published in 1966 because it is still useful in its original form. There are three pages in the beginning of Chapter 1 that depict the quandary of researchers in schizophrenia that are no longer accurate. Since the discovery of the role of the neurotransmitters in pain transmission, researchers who investigate the bodily aspects of schizophrenia and the other major mental illnesses believe that they

ix

are now asking the right questions and that knowledge of the causes and cures of the major mental illnesses will be uncovered within their own lifetimes. This research, which grew out of the use of tranquilizers, has also convinced many psychiatrists that tranquilizers not only are important in the treatment of mental illness but also hold the key to the understanding and conquest of these problems. These are heady times for somatic theories of mental illness. I must point out that although their hypothesis is credible, it remains a hypothesis. To date, there has been no demonstrable link between neurotransmission and mental illness. The idea that the mentally ill suffer from deficient or excessive neurotransmission is only a theory. Furthermore, even if the connection were made, most of the basic issues involving the social control of mental illness would remain. Since the connection is still hypothetical, it is premature to discard the labeling theory of mental illness.

The same reasoning applies to what has been called the "tranquilizer revolution." As Chapter 11 makes clear, even the most useful of the tranquilizers do not cure mental illness—they alleviate the symptoms. And again, even if a drug treatment were found that could cure mental illness, the fundamental issues of social control would remain. When the painkilling properties of morphine were discovered, physicians called it "God's Own Medicine" because they thought it was a cure. It took many years to realize that it was only a painkiller. There may be a parallel to be drawn between the discovery of morphine and that of tranquilizers. It has only been 28 years since the large-scale use of tranquilizers began. It may still be too early to evaluate their overall effects.

I am not arguing that the neurotransmitter hypothesis is incorrect, or that tranquilizers are worthless; I am only suggesting that it is much too early to discard the labeling theory of mental illness, despite the significant gains that have been made. Some balance is required in evaluating the competing claims of both the somatic and the social theorists. In recent years, there has been a tendency in sociology to overstate the claims of labeling theory. To avoid this overstatement, I have made two changes in the text. First, I have relinquished the "single most important" phrase in Proposition 9, stating instead that labeling is among the most important causes. The issue of the order of importance of the various causes is empirical anyway and should not have been reduced to a theoretical claim. The second change involves qualifying the contrast between the two poles of the societal reaction. Originally, I called the reaction to deviance that was opposite to labeling "denial"; in this edition I have changed it to "normalization." In fact, denial is only one of many differing ways of reacting to deviance, such as rationalization, ignoring, and temporizing. In the context of mental illness it is important to note that treatment is not necessarily a labeling reaction. Humane treatment may also be a form of normalization.

It is my hope that this edition in its expanded form will provide a clear statement of a purely sociological approach to mental illness.

Thomas J. Scheff

ACKNOWLEDGMENTS

SUPPORT for the writing of this book was provided by the following: the Graduate Research Committee of the University of California, Santa Barbara; the Social Science Research Council; and the Center for the Study of Law and Society, University of California, Berkeley.

Parts of the text have appeared earlier as articles: "The Social Role of the Mentally Ill and the Dynamics of Mental Disorder: A Research Framework," *Sociometry* 26 (December 1963): 436–453 (parts of Chapters 3 and 4); "Social Supports for Stereotypes of Mental Illness," *Mental Hygiene* 47 (July 1963): 461–469 (part of Chapter 4); "Decision Rules, Types of Error, and their Consequences in Medical Diagnosis," *Behavioral Science* 8 (April 1963): 97–107 (part of Chapter 5); "The Societal Reaction to Deviance: Ascriptive Elements in the Psychiatric Screening of Mental Patients in a Midwestern State," *Social Problems* 11 (Spring, 1964): 401–413 (Study 1 in Chapter 6). Some of the data presented in Study II, Chapter 6, were described in "Legitimate, Transitional, and Illegitimate Mental Patients in a Midwestern State," *American Journal of Psychiatry* 120 (September 1963): 267–269; and "Typification in Diagnosis," *Sociology and Rehabilitation,* in Marvin B. Sussman (ed.), American Sociological Association, Washington, D.C. (1965): 139–147, contains parts of Chapter 5. "Users and Nonusers of a Student Psychiatric Clinic," *Journal of Health and Human Behavior* 7 (1966): 114–121 (Chapter 7); "Negotiating Reality: Notes on Power in the Assessment of Responsibility," *Social Problems* 16 (1968): 3–17 (Chapter 8); "The Stability of Deviant Behavior over Time: A Reassessment," *Journal of Health and Social Behavior* 11 (1970): 37–43; "On Reason and Sanity: Some Political Implications of Psychiatric Thought," in William Lebra (ed.), *Culture and Mental Health in the Pacific,* The University Press of Hawaii, Honolulu (1972): 400–406 (Chapter 10); "Medical Dominance: Psychoactive Drugs and Mental Health Policy," *American Behavioral Scientist* 19 (1976): 299–317 (Chapter 11); "The Labeling Theory of Mental Illness," *American Sociological Review* 39 (1974): 444–452 (Chapter 12); "The Labeling Theory

Paradigm," in Carl Eisdorfer, Donna Cohen, Arthur Kleinman, and Peter Maxim (eds.), *Models for Clinical Pathology,* SP Medical and Scientific Books, New York (1981): 27–41 (Chapter 13).

Permission to republish these articles in revised form is gratefully acknowledged to these journals.

I wish to acknowledge the help of the following persons: Sarah Bradly composed and drew the montage and flow chart in Chapter 4; Walter Buckley gave helpful advice on theory and systems; Howard Becker, Arlene Daniels, and Tamotsu Shibutani read earlier drafts and gave editorial advice concerning the first edition. Needless to say, the errors and inconsistencies in this book are entirely my responsibility.

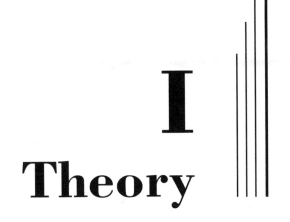

I
Theory

Introduction:
Individual and Social Systems
in Deviance

1

ALTHOUGH the last five decades have seen a vast number of studies of functional mental disorder, there is as yet no substantial, verified body of knowledge in this area.[1] At this writing, there is no rigorous knowledge of the cause, cure, or even the symptoms of functional mental disorders. Such knowledge as there is, is clinical and intuitive, and thus not subject to verification by scientific methods.

Consider, for example, the research that has been done on the origins of schizophrenia, one of the major mental disorders. Lewis (1936) reports that from 1920 to 1934, 1778 papers, monographs, and books were published on organic studies of schizophrenia. For the period from 1935 to 1945, Bellak (1948) counted 3200 studies on this subject. Finally, for the period 1940–1960, Jackson (1960) counted some 500 papers on etiology alone. Even allowing for the overlap between Bellak's and Jackson's reports, we can estimate that there have been at least 5000 papers reporting research on schizophrenia in the five decades since 1920.

What progress has been made as a result of this massive investigation of schizophrenia? Arieti (1955) summarizes the results of the organic studies: "The quantity of these works and the variety of directions which they have taken reveal that no headway has been made and that no constructive avenue of research has

[1]See Preface for a note about these first three pages of text.

3

yet been found in the organic field. [p. 9]." Jackson (1960), summarizing the later papers, states:

> These papers disagree widely with one another and reflect the fact that schizophrenia is a singularly difficult disorder to investigate. . . .
>
> At present, schizophrenia is one of our major medical problems. This is not only because of its incidence (estimated at from one to three per cent of the population) and its chronicity (keeping one quarter of the hospital beds in the country occupied), or because of the fact that its major incidence is during the most productive periods of life, roughly between the ages of 15 and 44. *It is also because medicine has made progress against many other major disorders, thus allowing schizophrenia to loom large by contrast* [pp. 3–4; emphasis added].

In other words, Jackson is saying that virtually no progress has been made in research on schizophrenia.

The enormous outpouring of time and effort in the study of schizophrenia and the insignificant findings from this effort have caused considerable concern among psychiatric researchers. Many of these researchers have suggested that what is needed is not only more research but research which departs radically from the framework in which these earlier studies were made. A quotation from a recent symposium on schizophrenia suggests the need for a fundamental shift in perspective: "During the past decade, the problems of chronic schizophrenia have claimed the energy of workers in many fields. Despite significant contributions which reflect continuing progress, *we have yet to learn to ask ourselves the right questions* [Apter, 1960; emphasis added]." Many investigators, not only in the field of schizophrenia, but from all the studies of functional mental disorder, apparently now agree; not only have systematic studies failed to provide answers to the problem of causation, but there is considerable feeling that the problem itself has not been formulated correctly.

One frequently noted deficiency in psychiatric formulations of the problem is the failure to incorporate social processes into the dynamics of mental disorder. Although the importance of these processes is increasingly recognized by psychiatrists, the conceptual models used in formulating research questions are basically concerned with individual rather than social systems. Genetic, biochemical, and psychological investigations seek different causal agents but utilize similar models: dynamic systems that are located within the individual. In these investigations, social processes tend to be relegated to a subsidiary role, because the model focuses attention on individual differences rather than on the social system in which the individual is involved.

Even in the theories that are not organic in nature, the social system is relegated to a relatively minor place in the understanding of mental illness. This is true in psychoanalytic theory, the most influential of the nonorganic theories, although Freud and his students frequently noted the importance of the social and cultural setting. In order to underscore the importance of the system properties of a theory, it is useful to compare psychoanalytic ideas, which are built around individual systems, with Marxist analysis, which is entirely social systemic and excludes completely any consideration of individual systems.

In psychoanalytic theory, the origins of neurosis are external to the individual. Freud's formulation was: "The Oedipus complex is the kernel of every neurosis." Fenichel, Freud's disciple and chief codifier of psychoanalytic ideas, states: "The Oedipus complex is the normal climax of infantile sexual development as well as the basis of all neuroses [1945:108]." According to this theory, all children pass through a stage in which the parent of the opposite sex is chosen as a sexual object, causing intense hostility and rivalry toward the parent of the same sex. For children who go on to become normal adults, the Oedipal conflict is resolved: the child rejects the opposite-sex parent as a sexual object and identifies with the parent of his same sex. The rejection of his parent as a sexual object frees him from later incestuous and therefore guilt-laden sexual impulses, and the identification with the same-sex parent begins the formation of the super-ego, which is the very basis for a normal adult psychic structure.

If, however, the opposite-sex parent is not rejected as a sex object and the same-sex parent not taken as a model, a fundamental fault is created in the psychic structure. In this case, the person grows into an adult who is never psychologically separated from his parents: Throughout his life, he is fighting and refighting the Oedipal conflict. All his relations with persons of the opposite sex are tinged with incestuous guilt, because his perceptions are based on his early childhood images in the family. Similarly, all his relations with same-sex persons are colored by the hostility and rivalry he felt for his parent of the same sex. According to this theory, the boy who goes through childhood without resolving the Oedipal conflict never establishes new relationships with women or men in later life but is imprisoned within the incestuous, and therefore psychologically untenable, relationship with his mother, and the hostile, rivalry-ridden relationship with his father.

Fenichel notes that the social situation in the child's family at the time of the Oedipal conflict is a key determinant of whether the conflict is resolved. The absence of the one of the parents, or the weakness of one or the other as a model, as well as many other contingencies, are potential causes of lack of resolution. It should be noted, however, that these external sources of defect are no longer involved in the neurotic system of behavior after the Oedipal stage passes (approximately from the ages of 3–7 years). If the Oedipal conflict is not resolved at this stage, the psychic flaw will continue throughout later life, more or less independently of later life experiences. It is true that psychoanalysts do speak of precipitating factors in adult life, but it is clear that these factors are of only subsidiary interest. The person in the throes of the Oedipal conflict is a defective adult, such that stresses that others could easily surmount may plunge him into a full-scale neurosis.

Thus the psychoanalytic model of neurosis is basically a system of behavior that is contained within the individual. The external situation in which the individual is involved is seen only as an almost limitless source of triggers for a fully developed neurotic conflict within the individual. Psychoanalytic theory, like most contemporary theories of mental illness, whether they are psychological or organic, locates the neurotic system within the individual. To be sure, psychoanalysts, like other psychiatric theorists, allow for external causation. Fenichel (1945) states:

> The normal person has few "troops of occupation" remaining at the position "Oedipus complex," to use Freud's metaphor, the majority of his troops having marched on. However, under *great* duress they, too, may retreat, and thus a normal person may become neurotic. The person with a neurotic disposition has left nearly all his forces at the Oedipus complex; only a few have advanced, and at the slightest difficulty they have to go back and rejoin the main force at their first stand, the Oedipus complex [p. 108].

Similar disclaimers can be found in virtually all the current theories of mental illness. Needless to say, in these theories, as in psychoanalytic theory, the direction and thrust of the perspective is found not in these exceptions and qualifications, but in systemic linkages that they posit, connecting key characteristics of individuals with their neurotic behavior. In psychoanalytic theory, the great conceptual development occurs in linking the origins of neurosis in the Oedipal stage through the mechanisms of psychosexual development to their end result, which is treated by the psychoanalyst theoreticians in a great wealth of detail: the formations of dreams, everyday slips and errors, and finally, in their manifold variety and complexity, the neurotic symptoms.

Many of the critics of psychoanalytic theory have focused on just this feature as objectionable: the tracing of the most diverse kinds of human reactions back to the generic psychological substructure resulting from the Oedipal conflict. Freud's critics claim that the psychoanalytic model of man is too tight, narrow, rigid, and one-dimensional. The way in which psychoanalysts have sought to show how artistic creativity derives from psychosexual conflict is a case in point. Critics have also objected to Freud's key postulate of the "overdetermination" of symptoms. The literature of psychoanalysis abounds in instances showing how a symptom is not simply a consequence of a single cause but is merely one aspect of a veritable network of psychic phenomena. It is for this reason that psychoanalysts are usually adverse to the treatment of symptoms: their theory leads them to expect that if a symptom is removed, without changing the basic psychological structure, a new symptom will shortly appear in its place. But critics have objected that psychoanalytic theory seems to posit a type of pre-destination in which the neurotic is prisoner of his inexorable neurotic system.

From the point of view of the construction of a viable scientific theory, however, much of this criticism seems misplaced. It is just the "systemness" of psychoanalytic theory that makes it such a powerful intellectual weapon for the investigation of neurotic behavior. Starting from relatively few general postulates, it develops an enormous number of propositions about very concrete types of behavior. Such a theory is both powerful, in that it ramifies into many areas of behavior, and at least potentially refutable, so that with an adequate program of empirical research it could be qualified, transformed, or rejected.

Furthermore, the notion of the "overdetermination" of symptoms is very much in accord with recent developments in theory construction. In general systems theory, for example, the idea of overdetermination is closely related to the model of a self-maintaining system. The key feature of such a system is "negative feedback," such that deviations from the system's steady state are detected and fed back into the system in such a way as to cause the system to return to its steady state. There is no reason to believe that such a system is found in only biological or electronic realms; psychoanalytic interpretations have suggested many ways in which psychological systems have this property. In the discussion in the following chapters, a system with self-maintaining properties composed of the deviant and those reacting to him will be delineated.

The objection to psychoanalytic theory that is made here is not that it posits neurotic behavior as part of a closed system, but that the system that it formulates is too narrow, in that it leaves out aspects of the social context that are vital for understanding mental disorder. The basic model upon which psychoanalysis is constructed is the disease model, in that it portrays neurotic behavior as unfolding relentlessly out of a defective psychological system that is entirely contained within the body. To bring the individual systemic character of psychoanalytic theory into high relief, it is instructive to contrast it with Marxian theory, which is social systemic.

Like Freud, Marx began his analysis with relatively few, but highly abstract, postulates. Chief among these postulates is the dictum that in any society it is the mode of production that determines the basic social forms, including the economic and political systems, the direction and pace of social change, and, ultimately, even man's consciousness. This point is made very clearly when Marx states that the mode of production is the substructure and all other forms mere superstructure in any society. Marx went on to construct from this basic premise a theory of history and of society in which the characteristics of individuals are more or less irrelevant.

In his analysis of then contemporary Europe, Marx posited the accumulation of capital as the process that determined social structure and social change. In primitive capitalism, the critical step was the accumulation of sufficient captial that a man's subsistence was not continually in jeopardy. The early capitalist could afford to bargain for his labor rather than accept whatever the market offered. Society was transformed into two classes, those in a bargaining position (the capitalists) and those who were not (the workers). In the course of bargaining, the market rates for labor inevitably assumed the bottom limit, the cost of the worker's subsistence, and the capitalists, by the same logic, inevitably waxed rich at the worker's expense. For our purposes, the interesting feature of Marx's theory was the manner in which it disregarded the motivations of the individuals involved. For the capitalists, for example, it did not matter whether they were humanitarian or not for the development of the capitalist system. A capitalist, who, for humane reasons, refused to expropriate the workers, would himself be expropriated by other capitalists. Marx and his followers felt that they had evolved a theory that was independent of the psychology of individuals.

From these considerations, Marx (1906) stated the law of capital accumulation:

> But all methods for the production of surplus value are at the same time methods of accumulation; and every extension of accumulation becomes again a means for the development of those methods. It follows therefore that in proportion as capital accumulates, the lot of the laborer, be his payment high or low, must grow worse. The law, finally, that always equilibrates the relative surplus-population, or industrial reserve army, to the extent and energy of accumulation, this law rivets the laborer to capital more firmly than the wedges of Vulcan did Prometheus to the rock. It established an accumulation of misery, corresponding with accumulation of capital. Accumulation of wealth at one pole is, therefore, at the same time accumulation of misery, agony of toil, slavery, ignorance, brutality, and mental degradation, at the other pole [pp. 708–709].

Marx (1906) notes the social and psychological effect of this process on the individual laborer:

> Within the capitalist system all methods for raising the social productiveness of labor are brought about at the cost of the individual laborer; all means for the development of production transform themselves into domination over, and exploitation of, the producers; they mutilate the laborer into a fragment of a man, degrade him to the level of an appendage of a machine, destroy every remnant or charm in his work and turn it into a hated toil; they estrange from him the intellectual potentialities of the labor process in the same proportion as science is incorporated in it as an independent power; they distort the conditions under which he works, subject him during the labor process to a depotism the more hateful for its meanness; they transform his life-time to a working time, and drag his wife and child beneath the wheels of the Juggernaut of capital [p. 708].

Beginning with the dynamics of the economic system, Marx developed propositions that lead finally to a prediction of psychological consequence for individuals. The statement concerning estrangement from the intellectual potentialities of labor, together with other similar statements, is one basis for current formulations about alienation, a psychological condition that is one of the subjects of recent psychiatric discussion.

For the purposes of this discussion, the failures of Marxian theory are not as important as the general form it takes. The rise of effective industrial unions vitiated Marx's analysis near its premise, the irreversibility of the law of capital accumulation. The form of his theory, however, provides an example of a social systemic model that does not include any aspects of individual systems of behavior. The question raised by this comparison is this: can we formulate a theory which somehow integrates both the individual and social systems of behavior?

Recently, a number of writers have begun to develop an approach that gives more emphasis to social processes than does traditional psychiatric theory yet does not neglect entirely individual aspects. Lemert (1951), Erikson (1957), and

Goffman (1961), among sociologists, and Szasz (1961) and Laing and Esterson (1964), among psychiatrists, have contributed notably to this approach. Lemert, particularly, by rejecting the more conventional concern with the origins of mental symptoms and stressing instead the potential importance of the societal reaction in stabilizing rule-breaking, focuses primarily on mechanisms of social control. The work of all these authors suggests research avenues that are analytically separable from questions of individual systems and point, therefore, to a theory that would incorporate social processes.

In his discussion of gamesmanship, Berne (1964) offers an analysis of alcoholism that is based on a social system model rather than on an individual system model of alcoholism:

> In game analysis there is no such thing as alcoholism or ''an alcoholic,'' but there is a role called the Alcoholic in a certain type of game. If a biochemical or physiological abnormality is the prime mover in excessive drinking—and that is still open to some question—then its study belongs in the field of internal medicine. Game analysis is interested in something quite different—the kinds of social transactions that are related to such excesses. Hence the game ''Alcoholic.''
>
> In its full flower this is a five-handed game, although the roles may be condensed so that it starts off and terminates as a two-handed one. The central role is that of the Alcoholic—the one who is ''it''—played by White. The chief supporting role is that of Persecutor, typically played by a member of the opposite sex, usually the spouse. The third role is that of Rescuer, usually played by someone of the same sex, often the good family doctor who is interested in the patient and also in drinking problems. In the classical situation the doctor successfully rescues the alcoholic from his habit. After White has not taken a drink for six months they congratulate each other. The following day White is found in the gutter.
>
> The fourth role is that of the Patsy, or Dummy. In literature this is played by the delicatessen man who extends credit to White, gives him a sandwich on the cuff and perhaps a cup of coffee, without either persecuting him or trying to rescue him. In life this is more frequently played by White's mother, who gives him money and often sympathizes with him about the wife who does not understand him. In this aspect of the game, White is required to account in some plausible way for his need for money—by some project in which both pretend to believe, although they know what he is really going to spend most of the money for. Sometimes the Patsy slides over into another role, which is a helpful but not essential one: the Agitator, the ''good guy'' who offers supplies without even being asked for them: ''Come have a drink with me (and you will go downhill faster).''
>
> The ancillary professional in all drinking games is the bartender or liquor clerk. In the game ''Alcoholic'' he plays the fifth role, the Connection, the direct source of supply who also understands alcoholic talk, and who in a way is the most meaningful person in the life of any addict. The difference between the Connection and the other players is the difference between professionals and amateurs in any game: the professional knows when to stop. At a certain point a good bartender refuses to serve the Alcoholic, who is then left without any supplies unless he can locate a more indulgent Connection [pp. 73–74].

Berne seems to be suggesting that the dynamics of alcoholism have less to do with the motivations and traits of the alcoholic than with the interactions between the occupants of the five interpersonal positions that he describes. According to his analysis, alcohol behavior is understandable only as an integral part of an interpersonal system.

A critique of the use of the medical model in psychiatry that parallels many aspects of the present discussion has been made by learning theorists in psychology. A thorough and well-documented statement can be found in the introduction to *Case Studies in Behavior Modification* (Ullman and Krasner, 1965). The psychological model that is proposed as an alternative to the medical model is based on the stimulus–response arc. The resultant processes of diagnosis and treatment have been described simply by Eysenck (1959): "Learning theory does not postulate any such "unconscious cause," but regards neurotic symptoms as simple learned habits; there is no neurosis underlying the symptom, but merely the symptom itself. *Get rid of the symptom and you have eliminated the neurosis.* [pp. 61–75; quoted in Ullman and Krasner, 1965]. The approach to mental disorder proposed by these researchers appears to be superior to the medical model in three ways: First, it is behavioral and therefore allows for empirical research. Second, it is related to a systematic and explicitly stated body of propositions (i.e., learning theory). Finally, it is supported by a sizeable body of empirical studies. It seems clear that this approach has made important contributions to psychiatric theory and practice and is likely to lead to fruitful work in the future.

At the same time, it should also be noted that "behavior modification," in practice, tends to be used as an individual system model of mental disorder. Conceptually, this is not necessarily the case. Ullmann and Krasner conceptualize psychiatric symptoms as maladaptive behavior. They go on to say that the goal of treatment of maladaptive behavior should be to change the patient's relationship to environmental stimuli. This formulation does not prejudge the question of whether the relationship should be changed by changing the patient or the environment. But in listing the techniques used in behavior modification, it is clear that the target for these techniques is the patient. Such techniques as "assertive responses, sexual responses, relaxation responses, conditioned avoidance responses, feeding responses, chemotherapy, expressive therapy, emotive imagery, *in vivo* presentation of disruptive stimuli, modeling, negative practice, self-disclosure, extinction, selective positive reinforcement, and stimulus deprivation and satiation" are the major techniques listed by Ullmann and Krasner. These techniques are oriented toward changing the patient's psychological system rather than the interpersonal or social system of which he is a member. Furthermore, it is not clear how it is possible for the therapist to effect changes through conditioning when in actual fact the technique utilized by the therapist constitutes only a small fraction of the total environmental stimulation to which the patient is exposed.

Like the medical model, "behavior modification" tends to isolate the symptom from the context in which it occurs. This occurs even in carefully formulated statements such as the following of Ullmann and Krasner (1965). In their statement, they are very careful to relate maladaptive behavior to the social context:

> Maladaptive behaviors are learned behaviors, and the development and maintenance of a
> maladaptive behavior is no different from the development and maintenance of any other

behavior. There is no discontinuity between desirable and undesirable modes of adjustment or between "healthy" or "sick" behavior. The first major implication of this view is the question of how a behavior is to be identified as desirable or undesirable, adaptive or maladaptive. The general answer we propose is that because there are no disease entities involved in the majority of subjects displaying maladaptive behavior, the designation of a behavior as pathological or not is dependent upon the individual's society [p. 20].

To this point, their formulation concerning "maladaptive behavior" exactly parallels the definition of deviant behavior presented here. They go on to further specify the meaning of maladaptive behavior in terms of roles and role reinforcement.

Specifically, while there are no single behaviors that would be said to be adaptive in all cultures, there are in all cultures definite expectations or roles for functioning adults in terms of familial and social responsibility. Along with role enactments, there are a full range of expected potential reinforcements. The person whose behavior is maladaptive does not fully live up to the expectations for one in his role, does not respond to all the stimuli actually present, and does not obtain typical or maximum forms of reinforcement available to one of his status. . . . Maladaptive behavior is behavior that is considered inappropriate by those key people in a person's life who control reinforcers [p. 20].

Restated in sociological terms, their formulation is that deviance is the violation of social norms and leads to negative social sanctions. Again, the parallel between the psychological and the sociological formulation is quite close.

This formulation of maladaptive behavior in terms of role expectations and reinforcement is potentially a powerful psychological tool, since it tends to bring in the mechanisms of social control and provides a strong link, therefore, between individual and social system models of behavior. To maintain this link, however, it is necessary to remember that the classification of behavior as maladaptive is made relative to the standards of some particular society and is not an absolute judgment. (The same reasoning is applicable, of course, to the concept of *deviance*.)

It appears to be very difficult to maintain a relativistic stance when the individual system models are used, particularly when the framework is transmitted to students. An instance of this difficulty is represented by the work of Sullivan and his students. Although Sullivan sought to take psychiatric symptoms out of the patient by defining them as disorders of interpersonal relationships, his students put them back in by defining mental illness as a deficiency in the *capacity* for interpersonal relations. This individualization of social system concepts can be seen in the Ullmann and Krasner formulation, when they define one criterion of maladaptive behavior as not responding to "all the stimuli actually present." Since the response to stimuli of anyone in any role is highly selective, it would seem that the definition at this point had reverted to the absolute definition of deviance in terms of individual pathology. One function of a social system model of mental disorder is to provide a framework for research which facilitates an approach to mental disorder which is free of the questionable assumptions of inherent pathology in psychiatric symptoms.

Of the formulations of anthropologists, the one which most nearly parallels the model described here is the biocultural model of Anthony F. C. Wallace (1961). Giving somewhat more emphasis to organic sources of rule-breaking, Wallace posits that the initial cause of mental illness is physiological, but that the cultural "mazeways" (cognitive maps) profoundly shape the course of illness. In some detail, he notes how the "theories" of illness of the sick individual, his family and associates, and the "professionals" impinge on illness as a behavior system. The chief components of a "theory" of illness are to be:

1. The specific *states* (normalcy, upset, psychosis, in treatment, and innovative personality).
2. The *transfer mechanisms* that explain (to the satisfaction of the member of the society) how the sick person moves from one state to another.
3. The *program* of illness and recovery that is described by the whole system.

Wallace gives an extended analysis of one particular syndrome, the Eskimo *pibloktoq*, an acute excitement sometimes known as Arctic hysteria. According to his theory, pibloktoq has a physiological base in calcium deficiency (hypocalcemia) but is shaped by the culture-bound interpretations made by the sick persons and those who deal with him. Following Wallace's model, Fogelson (1965) presents a detailed analysis of *windigo*, a syndrome of compulsive cannibalism reported among Northern Algonkian-speaking Indians, which emphasizes culture-bound interpretations of rule-breaking behavior. The relationship between Wallace's model and the model developed here will be discussed later (Chapter 6).

The purpose of the present discussion is to state a set of nine propositions which make up basic assumptions for a social system model of mental disorder. This set is largely derived from the work of Wallace and Fogelson; all but two of the propositions (Nos. 4 and 5) being suggested, with varying degrees of explicitness, in the cited references. By stating these propositions explicitly, this theory attempts to facilitate testing of basic assumptions, all of which are empirically unverified or only partly verified. By stating these assumptions in terms of standard sociological concepts, the relevance to studies of mental disorder of findings from diverse areas of social science, such as race relations and prestige suggestion are shown. This theory also delineates three problems which are crucial for a sociological theory of mental disorder: what are the conditions in a culture under which diverse kinds of rule-breaking become stable and uniform; to what extent, in different phases of careers of mental patients, are symptoms of mental illness the result of conforming behavior; is there a general set of contingencies which lead to the definition of deviant behavior as a manifestation of mental illness? Finally, this discussion attempts to formulate special conceptual tools which are directly linked to sociological theory to deal with these problems.

The social institution of insanity, residual rule-breaking, deviance, the social role of the mentally ill, and the bifurcation of the societal reaction into the alternative reactions of denial and labeling are examples of such conceptual tools.

These conceptual tools are utilized to construct a theory of mental disorder in which psychiatric symptoms are considered to be labeled violations of social norms and stable "mental illness" to be a social role. The validity of this theory depends upon verification of the nine propositions listed in future studies and should, therefore, be applied with caution and with appreciation for its limitations. One such limitation is that the theory attempts to account for a much narrower class of phenomena than is usually found under the rubric of mental disorder; the discussion that follows will be focused exclusively on stable or recurring mental disorder and does not explain the causes of single episodes. A second major limitation is that the theory probably distorts the phenomena under discussion. Just as the individual system models understress social processes, the model presented here probably exaggerates their importance. The social system model "holds constant" individual differences in order to articulate the relationship between society and mental disorder. Ultimately, a framework which encompassed both individual and social systems and distorted the contribution of neither would be desirable. Given the present state of formulations in this area, this framework may prove useful by providing an explicit contrast to the more conventional medical and psychological approaches and thus assist in the formulation of socially oriented studies of mental disorder.

It should be made clear at this point that the purpose of this theory is *not* to reject psychiatric and psychological formulations in their totality. It is obvious that such formulations have served, and will continue to serve, useful functions in theory and practice concerning mental illness. The author's purpose, rather, is to develop a model which will complement the individual system models by providing a complete and explicit contrast. Although the individual system models of mental disorder have led to gains in research and treatment, they have also systematically obscured some aspects of the problem. The social system model, like the psychological model, highlights some aspects of the problem and obscures others. It does, however, allow a fresh look at the field, since the problems it clarifies are apt to be those that are most obscure when viewed from the psychiatric or medical point of view.

The case for the use of limited analytic models was clearly stated by Max Weber (1949), for analysis which he called "one-sided":

> The justification of the one-sided analysis of cultural reality from specific "points of view" . . . emerges purely as a technical expedient from the fact that training in the observation of the effects of qualitatively similar categories of causes and the repeated utilization of the same scheme of concepts and hypotheses offers all the advantages of the division of labor. It is free of the charge of arbitrariness to the exent that it is successful in producing insights into inter-connections which have been shown to be valuable in the causal explanation of concrete historical events [p. 71; quoted by Mechanic, 1963:167].

It can be argued that in addition to the advantages of the division of scientific labor as suggested by Weber, there is yet another advantage to one-sided analysis. In the nature of scientific investigation, a central goal is the development of the "crucial experiment," a study whose results allow for the decisive comparison of two opposing theories, such that one is upheld and the other rejected. Implicit in the goal of the crucial experiment is the conception of science as an adversarial process in which scientific progress arises out of the confrontation of explicitly conflicting theories. In his formulation of the history of change in the natural sciences, Kuhn (1962) considers all scientific progress as the conflict between "competing paradigms" (i.e., opposing theories). Whitehead has stated this view very clearly: "A class of doctrines is not a disaster—it is an opportunity. . . . In formal logic, a contradiction is the signal of a defeat; but in the evolution of real knowledge it marks the first step in progress towards a victory [pp. 266–267]."

One road of progress in science is the intentional formulation of mutually incompatible models, each incomplete and each explicating only a portion of the area under investigation. The advance of science, as in the theory of adversarial procedures in law, rests on the dialectical process which occurs when incommensurate positions are placed in conflict. In the present discussion of mental illness, the social system model is proposed not as an end in itself but as the antithesis to the individual system model. By allowing for explicit consideration of these antithetical models, the way may be cleared for a synthesis, a model which has the advantages of both the individual and the social system models but the disadvantages of neither.

In the discussion that follows Part I, a sociological theory of mental illness first will be developed. The theory, in turn, provides the framework for the field studies which are reported in the later part of the book. The theory has two basic components: social role and the societal reaction. Its key assumptions are that most chronic mental illness is at least in part a social role, and that the societal reaction is usually the most important determinant of entry into that role. Throughout Part I the discussion that follows, this sociological model will continually be compared with and contrasted with the more conventional medical and psychological models of mental illness in an attempt to delineate significant problems for further analysis and research.

Part I of this book, in addition to this introduction, has three other chapters concerned with the statement of the theory of mental illness. Chapter 2 provides the background for Part I: a statement of the fundamental sociological notion of social control as a system. This chapter introduces Chapter 3, which is devoted to the basic premise of the theory: symptoms of mental illness are violations of residual rules. In this analysis, "mental illness' is considered, therefore, as residual deviance. Discussion of propositions concerning the origins, prevalence, and duration and consequences of residual deviance are found in this chapter.

In Chapter 4, "The Social Institution of Insanity," the rest of the theory is outlined. The first two sections of the chapter concern the social role of the mentally ill: how and why the role is played and the source of the role imagery in ordinary language and in the mass media. The last two sections of the chapter deal with the social system and its relation to deviant careers. This section contains a discussion of the part played by the societal reaction to rule breaking in causing or blocking entry into the role and status of the mentally ill. The final section describes the entire theory as a model in which the rule-breaking acts, the responses of others, and the rule-breaker's responses to these responses and so on are seen as constituting a system with definite boundaries and self-maintaining properties. The discussion of the social system model completes Part I.

Part II describes several studies that I conducted that were based on the theory outlined in Part I and that provide, in turn, support for certain aspects of the theory. In Chapter 5 the problem of uncertainty in diagnosis and the physician's reaction to uncertainty is explored. It is suggested that physicians tend to follow the rule, "when in doubt, diagnose illness, rather than health." Some of the implications and consequences of this rule are then discussed.

In Chapter 6, two field studies are reported that show how crucial the problem of the physician's response to uncertainty becomes in the handling of mental patients. The first study concerns the decision to hospitalize and treat; the second study considers the decision to release. Both studies provide very strong support for one of the central theses of the book: At the present time, the variables that afford the best understanding and prediction of the course of "mental illness" are not the refined etiological and nosological features of the illness but gross features of the community and legal and psychiatric procedures. (See Proposition 9 and the discussion that follows it in Chapter 4.)

The next three chapters also present studies with similar findings. Chapter 7 reports a study that surveyed the psychiatric symptoms of students who came to a psychiatric clinic on campus and a sample of the remaining students who did not use the clinic at all. Chapter 8 compares the tactics of a psychiatrist interviewing a client with those used by a defense lawyer with his client. Chapter 9 reviews prior studies of the duration of psychiatric symptoms over time.

Part III concerns two controversies connected with psychiatric theory. The first, Chapter 10, discusses the connection between psychiatric reasoning and political thought. Chapter 11 assesses the value of tranquilizers as a treatment for mental illness and the impact of having physicians in charge of the treatment of mental illness. Chapters 12 and 13 of Part IV review the state of evidence concerning labeling theory. Although the evidence is incomplete, it seems to suggest the value of labeling theory in a provisional way.

Chapter 14 explores some of the implications of the theory and research in the earlier chapters. The first section deals with the way in which behavior may or may not be seen as a psychiatric symptom, depending on the social context in which it occurs, and the preconceptions and procedures used by the diagnostician. Following from this discussion, a research proposal is outlined for making the diagnostic practices of health, custodial, and welfare organizations a subject for systematic research. The next section presents a description of the course of mental illness in terms of the structure and dynamics of social status: The distinction between sanity and insanity is depicted as a status system with many similarities to the "color line." This analysis raises a number of questions concerning theory and research and public policy.

The final section of Chapter 14 summarizes the argument and concludes the book. In the Appendix, a short explanation of the development and significance of the flow chart in Chapter 4 is provided by Walter Buckley.

Social Control as a System

2

Social scientists look at deviance in a somewhat different way from other members of the society. In order to understand *deviance* objectively (the sense in which I use this term will be defined shortly), they argue, one must first understand the more general phenomena of social control, the processes which generate conformity in human groups. This chapter introduces the theory of social control and shows how it applies to nondeviant areas such as clothing and appearance, language, facial expressions, feeling, and thought. Subsequent chapters demonstrate how this theory may be applied to the phenomenon of mental illness.

Rather than start the discussion of social control abstractly, I indicate some elements of social control in a concrete area, that of clothing and appearance. What determines the way people dress? In particular, why is there so much uniformity in dress within a given social group? We feel that we understand why soldiers wear uniforms, but why do corporation executives, sorority women, and college professors, for example? Perhaps one could explore his or her own choice of clothing. What determines one's style of dress or the choice of items in one's wardrobe? This may not be an easy question to answer. If that is the case, try reviewing the process that went into the choice of each particular garment. One may say, "I don't care what other people think, I dress to please myself." Even if it were true literally that one dresses only to please oneself, it is probably not true that the opinions of others have no impact at all. Some person's dress expresses the message: "I don't care what you think." Dressing to express this message betrays a form of social influence, if only a negative one. One may extend the exploration of the influences on one's appearance by reviewing how the significant people in one's life view your appearance. Such an exploration should reveal a great deal, not only about oneself but about the process of social control as it applies to oneself.

The social control of clothing has been evoked succinctly by Quentin Bell (1976):

> There is . . . a whole system of morality attached to clothes and more especially to fashion, a system different from and frequently at variance with that contained in our laws and our religion. To go to the theatre with five days' beard, to attend a ball in faultless evening dress . . . but with your braces outside, instead of within your white waistcoat, to scatter ink on your spats, to reverse your tie, these things are not incompatible with moral or theological teaching, the law takes no cognizance of such acts. Nevertheless such behaviour will excite the strongest censure in "good society," . . . it is not however sheer lunatic eccentricity such as the absence of trousers or a wig worn back to front which excites the strongest censure; far worse are those subtler forms of incorrect attire: the "wrong" tie, the "bad" hat, the "loud" skirt, the "cheap" scent, or the flamboyant checks of the overdressed vulgarian. Here the censure excited is almost exactly comparable to that occasioned by dishonourable conduct [p. 18].

Although some of the terms are English, the sentiments apply equally well to American society. In this excerpt, Bell makes an important point: nonconformity to community standards concerning appropriate dress can excite a very strong negative response from others. Furthermore, Bell notes, the community standards concerning clothing are not legal standards or religious standards. They may have no formal status at all. They seem to be unwritten or even, in some cases, unstated rules. Yet in spite of their informal status, they would appear to exert great influence over dress and appearance. This issue will be discussed later under the topic formal and informal norms.

Bell goes on to make a second important point about social control which concerns the relationship between individual and collective feelings with respect to dress:

> It is not simply the judgment of society which acts upon the individual. Our confusion when, having sat for two hours on the platform of a public meeting, we discover that we have been wearing odd socks, our still worse confusion when we find that our flies have been undone (even though nothing of any consequence has been revealed) has something of the quality of guilt. Indeed, I think it may frequently happen here, as in other moral situations, that the offender may be not simply the worst but in fact the only sufferer. A rebellious collar stud, a minute hole in a stocking may ruin an evening without ever being observed by the company at large. . . . "A sense of being perfectly well dressed," a lady is reported as saying to Emerson, "gives a feeling of inward tranquillity which religion is powerless to bestow" [p. 19].

Again, Bell makes an important point: The power of social control is not limited to the operation of *actual* censure but includes the operation of *imagined* censure. We all have suffered excruciating agonies of embarrassment in situations where the negative response of others to our appearance was mostly or even entirely in our imagination. Social control seldom operates so that individuals are passive recipients of other's responses: each person plays an active role both by imagining future responses of others and by defining present actions of others as responses to one's own behavior. Each individuals' actions both create and are created by social control. I will return to this idea shortly in the discussion of the part that self-control plays in social control.

In light of this discussion, a preliminary answer now can be given to the question concerning the uniformity in clothing that we see around us. Social control plays an important part in generating uniformity of dress and appearance. Social control involves the rewarding of conformity to shared expectations and the punishment of nonconformity. Clothing which conforms to the group standards of dress is rewarded with praise and admiration. If it does not conform, it is likely to generate criticism or disapproval.

The theory of social control is the major interpretive model in social science. It is for this reason that social scientists see deviance as a type of nonconformity and seek to understand deviance in terms of the operation of social control. This approach to deviance is distinctive to social science, separating it both from the view of laypersons, on the one hand, and from the experts on deviance like psychiatrists and police, on the other.

The social science approach to deviance is distinctive in three major ways. First, both laypersons and professionals who deal with deviants usually see deviance as mostly an individual matter, that is, they take an individual perspective toward deviance. What was it in the character and background of the deviant that caused him to become deviant? How can her deviance be stopped? Social scientists do not rule out these questions. But their framework is broader in that it deals both with the individual deviant and with societies' response. The individual perspective and the social control perspective are alternative ways of understanding deviance.

An example illustrates how the social control perspective is broader than the individual perspective. At a conference on child development, there was a discussion of the disruptive behavior of two ''hyperactive'' children in a class of 30 fifth-graders. The participants were focusing on the possible causes of the hyperactivity in the backgrounds of the children and the tactics that the teacher might use in managing their hyperactivity, including referral to a physician who might prescribe tranquilizing drugs. However, I had remembered that in initially describing the situation, the observer who had introduced the case had said that the teacher spoke in a monotone and was dull. I suggested that we might discuss a question alternative to the one on the table: what was wrong with the other 28 children that they also were not disruptive but tolerated dull and ineffective teaching? Although not all of the participants accepted my idea, it did lead to a restructuring of the discussion to include more of the larger context in which ''hyperactivity'' was taking place.

There are two distinctive ways of conceptualizing the sources of behavior: in the person or in the situation. Why don't my children do their homework? Perhaps because they are lazy. This answer puts the source of behavior in the children and ignores the context. An alternative answer would be because the homework is too difficult or too easy: they are not motivated by the task or the teacher. This answer puts the source of behavior in the context and ignores the children. Needless to say, any thoughtful analysis should allow for an examination of both the individuals and the context. Often the individual perspective on the sources of behavior is a somewhat disguised aspect of the naïve societal reaction: ignore the context, place the cause for deviance in negative traits inside the rule-breakers, and punish them. Dewey put the matter succinctly: "Give a dog a bad name and hang it."

There is a second major way in which the social science concept of *deviance* is distinctive. The concept of *deviance* itself is used in a dispassionate way, stripped of the opprobrium the word ordinarily carries. It means a violation of social norms which usually brings stigma and a strong negative reaction from others. Deviance is the violation of those rules which are felt to be worthy of high respect. Not all rule-breaking excites a negative reaction. In different times and places, the breaking of rules may be seen as innovative, creative, comical, or not worthy of notice. But when important emotionally weighted norms are broken, such as those upholding loyalty to one's country, strong feelings of outrage are usually mobilized. The violation of such norms is deviance in the sociological sense.

The sociologist, however, seeks to apply the term only in a relative sense: in a certain tribe, looking directly at the emperor's face is a deviant act—it causes outrage in the members of the tribe but not to the sociologist as an outsider. When the sociological concept of *deviance* is applied to one's own society, it requires an attitude of alienation, using the term *as if* it did not carry opprobrium to us, the users, but only to the other unself-conscious members of the society. The first lesson in this discussion is that sociological analysis can be alienating. It requires that the analyst be stationed outside of his / her own society.

Alienation is the sense that elements of one's own life are meaningless. Churchgoers sometims feel they are merely going through the motions of religion without any deeply felt conviction. Many students have similar reactions to their schooling, at least at times. At the opposite pole is the feeling of integration, of a powerful bond between one's inner feelings and outward behavior. [An exercise would be to recall experiences in one's own life of alienation and of integration.]

Stripping the word *deviant* of its heavy load of negative emotions may seem easy at first. When one realizes that it usually has extremely strong emotional connotations, then one can use the word in its neutral, sociological sense if one chooses. Actually, the emotional coloring is so strong and so complex that the stripping operation and the dispassionate use of the word is a difficult maneuver. As discussed shortly, we have all been socialized to feel extremely strong emotions toward deviance and deviants, profound reactions of resentment, fear, and embarrassment. These feelings usually cannot be completely controlled by the desire to be analytic and objective. The sociologist's intent to be dispassionate toward deviance exists in strong tension with his inclination to feel the negative emotions of his / her own tribe. Nevertheless, the sociological sense of deviance is still quite different from the ordinary sense of the idea, emotionally, since the tension between neutrality and emotional commitment itself is differentiating. The ordinary member of the tribe feels little or no tension in this respect: his / her condemnation of deviance is whole-hearted and unself-conscious. The sentiment behind "Lock them up in jail and throw away the key" is prevalent, even in those who would not openly endorse such a statement.

There is a third way in which the sociological use of the term deviance is different from the conventional usage. The sociological concept of deviance is embedded in a whole set of ideas about the larger system of which deviance is one part. Corresponding to each of these ideas is a set of terms, or nomenclature, for the various parts of the system. We have already used one of these other terms in the discussion, the concept of a *social norm*. Deviance is an aspect of a larger system which is composed of shared expectations, or norms, on the one hand, and sanctions (rewards and punishments), on the other. Systems of social control exert pressure for conformity to social norms through the operations of sanctions: conformity to shared expectations is rewarded, and nonconformity is punished.

Since the idea of social control provides this book with its principal focus, in the discussion that follows, I provide many examples of the operation of social control. Before doing so, however, I would like to discuss briefly two questions that the reader may have in encountering this argument: What is the purpose of this kind of analysis? The ideas proposed here are certainly awkward, and you say they may be alienating. Why isn't it possible to rely on the experts in our society for approaches to deviance? Professionals such as police and criminologists for crime and psychiatrists and clinical psychologists for mental disorder, drug use, and sexual deviance are in direct contact with the very deviants who are the subjects of this book. Their experience should justify their opinions.

My answer to these questions is in two parts. The first part is that one should not discard the findings and insights that are available in police science, criminology, psychiatry, and clinical psychology. This knowledge, as suggested in the question, is based on intimate and detailed knowledge of deviants and is, therefore, clearly of great value.

However, and this is a big however, I would also argue that although it is valuable, it is not enough by itself. There is an important bias in the collective wisdom of the professionals who regularly deal with deviants. In some important ways, these professionals are part of the system of social control that is described here. They are not entirely detached investigators of the process of deviance, since they themselves must deal with deviants in ways that are acceptable to the society. A policeman, warden, or clinical psychiatrist or psychologist who merely objectively studies clients would not last long in the job, since it calls, at least in part, for the enforcing of the appropriate social norms. The professionals who deal with deviance, because they are part of the system of social control, usually have a perspective which is, at least in part, congruent with the basic perspective of the particular society they represent. Most prison wardens or psychiatrists are not completely dispassionate about the crimes of their prisoners; they tend to see them, at least in part, as the society does, as abhorrent.

The social control framework offers a more detached and therefore, one hopes, more objective perspective for examining deviance and the control of deviance. This framework can be applied to deviance in any society, including the society of the analyst. As has already been mentioned, the dispassionate analysis of deviance in one's own society involves the analyst in conflict because of the very basic negative beliefs and feelings shared by all of the members of the society, including the social scientist. But conflict may heighten awareness. This heightening of awareness may be uncomfortable for the analyst but it also increases the objectivity and insightfulness of his / her analysis.

I now return to the concept of a *system of social control*. As indicated, this system is composed of a very large set of norms, on the one hand, and a set of sanctions, of punishments and rewards, which enforce the norms, on the other. I begin the discussion with a description of social norms. The simplest definition of a norm is a shared expectation, that is, an expectation that is shared by the members of a group. The sense in which an expectation is *shared* is rather complicated. Social norms can be incredibly rigid and impervious to change, but they can also change overnight. Paradoxically, norms can be both evanescent and unyielding. The great French sociologist, Durkheim, referred to them as *social facts*. It is instructive to compare these social facts with physical facts.

There is a sense in which a social fact is enormously more durable than the toughest physical material. The desert tribes which created the Ten Commandments have long since vanished; not a shard remains of their civilization. Yet the moral code they developed is very much alive today, part of the consciousness and behavior of those societies that have a Judeo-Christian heritage. The Ten Commandments survive not merely in the Bible but in our very lives and minds. Shared expectations of this kind are stronger than the strongest steel, more durable than gold.

As I have said, normative codes can collapse and vanish overnight. In any culture, panic and anarchy are unusual but not beyond possibility. More usually, definite change occurs in a measured or gradual way. Changes in shared expectations concerning clothing and appearance are an important part of the phenomena of fashion. Another example is the pervasive change in language over a much longer time period.

What is the nature of the process of sharing expectations such that norms can be either stronger than steel or weaker than gossamer? Furthermore, what is the relationship of individual expectations to those held by the group? In some instances, it is clear even to individuals strongly opposed to a norm that the norm exists, seemingly independently of their own will or the will of any persons whom they know. As Durkheim indicated, collective representations, or what we call here shared expectations, have exteriority and constraint. They may seem exterior to many or even most of the persons in the society where they obtain, and they are seen, therefore, as constraining on behavior: People actually feel pressure to conform. Durkheim (1963) sees norms as so powerful that he gives them a life of their own apart from the people who create them as "partially autonomous realities, with their own way of life." Durkheim does not actually answer the question raised here about the nature of the process involved in the creation and maintenance of shared expectations, he merely suggests that it occurs: "Collective representations are exterior to individual minds. . . . They do not derive from them as such, but from the association of minds, which is a very different thing."

How may one describe the details of the "the association of minds" that Durkheim refers to in a way which makes the exteriority and constraint of norms plausible? This is a crucial question for the understanding of social control. An answer has been suggested by the economist, Thomas Schelling. It is instructive to repeat an example he has given of the creation of a shared expectation, in this case, the understanding between the conflicting parties that the Yalu River was to be the boundary of the Korean War:

> If the Yalu River is to be viewed as a limit in the Korean War that was recognized on both sides, its force and authority is to be analyzed not in terms of the joint unilateral recognition of it by both sides of the conflict—not as something that we and the Chinese recognized unilaterally and simultaneously—but as something that we "mutually recognized." It was not just that we recognized it and they recognized it, but that we recognized that they recognized it, they recognized that we recognized it, we recognized that they recognized that we recognized it, and so on. It was a shared expectation. To that extent, it was a somewhat undeniable expectation. If it commands our attention, then we expect it to be observed and we expect the Chinese to expect us to observe it. We cannot unilaterally detach our expectations from it. In that sense limits and precedents and traditions of this kind have an authority that is not exactly granted to them voluntarily by the participants in a conflict. They acquire magnetism or focal power of their own [1963].

In this example, Schelling gives what I consider to be an extremely precise definition of a social norm. The people who come to share an expectation need not be in actual contact or consider themselves a group. In this case, the people are at war with each other. But they are sensitive to each other's gestures, so that they "mutually recognize" that they share an expectation. The sharing of the expectation is very deep in that it is not just that the parties all hold the expectation independently, but each recognizes that the other holds it, and each recognizes that the other recognizes that they hold it, and so on. The parties are not merely in agreement about the Yalu River, they are cooriented: "I know that you know that I know that if the United States forces go past the river, the Chinese Army will intervene." Another example: "I expect that others will not touch me intimately in public; I assume that most others share this expectation; I assume that most others assume that I share this expectation," etc. A shared expectation exists if there is an infinite series of reciprocating attributions between the members of the group.

As in my definition, Schelling allows for indefinitely high orders of reciprocating attribution. This allowance evokes Durkheim's exteriority and constraint in its final sentences:

> In that sense limits and precedents and traditions of this kind have an authority that is not exactly granted to them voluntarily by the participants in a conflict. They acquire magnetism or focal power of their own [1963].

The shared expectation is felt as a powerful exterior constraint because each individual agrees, recognizes that his neighbors agree, that they each recognize that he agrees, that he recognizes they recognize, and so on indefinitely. Although he agrees (or disagrees) with the sentiment, it is also something beyond his power to change, or even completely explore. The potentially endless mirror reflections of each of the others' recognitions is felt as something utterly final. From this formulation it follows that each actor feels the presence of expectation with a sense of exteriority and constraint, even if he, as an individual, is himself wholeheartedly dedicated or opposed to the expectation.

To each member of the society, therefore, norms appear to have both an inner reality, a sense of moral obligation and rectitude, and an outer reality, the sense that others are deeply and irrevocably involved in the same moral world as one's self.

The individual's sense of moral coercion from others is complexly determined, because it is, in part, an assumption, but it is also, in part, based on reality. One cannot help being aware that others are not indifferent to normative aspects of behavior. Even strangers, when in each other's presence, make subtle but forceful moral claims on each other. The temporary passengers in an elevator inhibit each other's behavior, even to the direction of glance. Most people feel compelled to look at the floor or elevator doors. These inhibitions arise because of actual or expected responses of others to one's behavior, as well as one's own sense of morality.

To put it in a slightly different way, the process of social control involves both control by others and self-control. Self-control operates in two related but different ways. First, the individual can imagine a whole world of response that may never occur. A female college student, considering whether to live with a male friend or not, may suddenly see the issue as her mother may see it—"What would mother think?" and be guided by her impression of her mother's judgment. Similarly, before standing up in front of the class and giving an answer to a question, a student may consider his answer not only from the professor's point of view but also from that of the class. In some instances, the student refrains from speaking, having imagined that his answer will seem ridiculous to one or both of these parties.

Second, even real actions of others must be interpreted by the individual as to whether they are responses to the individual's acts, that is, whether they are sanctions. As the student gives an answer in class, he notices that the professor is frowning. The student must decide if the professor's frown is a response to the student's answer. The student remembers that the professor was frowning before the question was asked and decides that the frown is not a response to the answer.

The student's interpretation is verified when the professor praises the answer. In the process of social control, sanctions are responses by other's to one's behavior. Social control involves imaginative rehearsal and / or interpretation and is, therefore, in part, a process of self-control.

Sanctions may be defined as responses that reward behavior which is seen as conforming to normative expectations (positive sanctions) or punish nonconforming behavior (negative sanctions). That is, they are responses to conformity which bring pleasure to the actor and to nonconformity which bring pain. The response need not be extreme and formal, as in the case of a long prison sentence for a major crime; it can be subtle and ephemeral—a frown directed at a speaker with a slight lisp. Social control exerts a powerful force over behavior because the sanctioning process is often continuous and seemingly automatic.

Social control is largely informal. In most instances, it goes on unstated, unseen, and unacknowledged. To be sure, there are important aspects of any system of social control that are formal and explicit. The legal system, both in its criminal and civil sections, as well as the disciplinary systems in organizations, function in a formal way as a part of social control. Laws, statutes, and codes may serve as explicitly stated norms, and fines, imprisonment, and other disciplinary procedures may serve as sanctions. But the overlap between these formal systems and the larger system of social control in which they serve a part is far from complete.

In the first place, the total system of social control in a society is vastly larger than all of the formal systems taken together. In any given society, the total number of laws and codes may be counted in the tens of thousands. The number of formal sanctions is usually extremely small, in the hundreds, perhaps. As suggested in the discussion of the areas of control, in which I consider, as examples, diverse areas such as clothing, language, facial expression, thought, and feeling, the tacit norms and sanctions may come to uncounted millions.

In the second place, the formal systems are not completely accurate indexes of the system of social control. All formal systems contain forms which are not part of functioning system of control—blue-stocking laws, for example, statutes that are unenforced, dead letter laws. The formal systems stand in relation to a system of social control as dictionaries and grammars stand to a living language: Formal description and usage overlap but are distinct entities.

AREAS OF SOCIAL CONTROL

A living language can be considered to arise out of the action of a pervasive system of social control. On the one hand, shared among the speakers are literally millions of expectations concerning grammar, syntax, pronunciation, inflection, gesture, and meaning. On the other hand, there is a continuous sanctioning process occurring, in which conformity is rewarded and nonconformity punished. In face-to-face conversation, it is customary for the listener to reward the speaker almost continuously for conformity by looking intently at the speaker, nodding one's head or making some other affirmative gesture, and by smiling or at least refraining from frowning. Each of these gestures is a means of communicating to the speaker: "You are doing fine. I am listening. I understand. Please continue." More abstractly, the listener is continually responding to the actions of the speaker with positive sanctions and, in the case of not frowning, with the absence of negative sanctions.

Violation of expectations regarding language, whether verbal or nonverbal, is usually met with misunderstanding or incomprehension at best. Often violations bring responses of ridicule or censure. Adults may censure each other's language violations subtly or diplomatically. Adults with children, or children with children, are much less restrained. The world of the stutterer or the lisper is usually a nightmare of embarrassment.

Group members are extraordinarily sensitive to even slight departures from normative speech expectations. Variations of speech which are extremely slight, such as those due to social class or regional background, will usually produce both real and imagined sanctions. Even a slight residue of working-class inflection from Boston or New Orleans will produce frowns of distaste among middle-class Californians.

As already indicated, clothing and outward physical appearance present another lesson in social control. In modern industrial societies, the rate of change of the fashion in clothing and appearance is much more rapid than fashion in language. Nevertheless, the system of control is equally relentless. As is frequently remarked, even the rebels against the harsh strictures of fashion soon establish their own system of control. The hippie rebellion of the 1960s, and the blue-jeaned, T-shirted adolescent of the 1970s quickly developed codes of their own as precise as the ones they rejected. For a teenager at the time of this writing, the choice of fabric, style, and color in buying a pair of Addidas may be a task requiring excruciating care.

Social control is exercised not only over clothing but over most other aspects of outward appearance. Hairstyling is an obvious case in point. The length of men's hair usually not only excites responses along an aesthetic dimension but also involves more momentous issues very quickly, as it did both in Cromwell's England and in the 1960s student movement, when it indicated political significance. The amount and style of facial cosmetics usually has analogous moral implications for women. In nineteenth-century America, for example, rouge and lipstick were the marks of actresses and prostitutes.

In most societies, fashion in appearance extends to the body itself. The amount of exposure of leg, buttocks, midriff, and bosom is rigidly monitored by custom. Even the shape of the body is not exempt; deformation of the body, especially the bodies of women, is regularly attempted through social control. Their feet have been bound and their lips and buttocks made to protrude by surgery in prior societies. In our own society, injections of silicone are used to shape, lift, and extend the breasts and buttocks, and surgery rejuvenates aging faces and necks. Normative body shapes are rewarded with admiration; non-normative shapes are punished with criticism or neglect.

The relentlessness and pervasiveness of social control over outward forms of behavior and appearance is easily described. But social control does not stop with outer forms; it penetrates deeply into the inner life of thought and feeling. I begin this discussion with the issue of control over facial expression, since facial expression partakes of both outer and inner worlds. There are many situations in which facial expression is clearly subject to social control. At a funeral or at a school examination, a smile may bring an open rebuke just as a frown may receive a similar response at a cocktail party. In the large cities in modern society, a norm governing facial expression in public appears to be developing: it requires an expression signaling no emotion. Some of the humor and apprehension generated by the film *Invasion of the Body Snatchers* rests on this issue: that the blankness of the zombies in the San Francisco locale only slightly exaggerates the behavior that is becoming the norm in real life.

The expectation that the public facial expression on a metropolitan street will be an emotionless mask presumably shows social control only over the outward expression of feeling. Often, however, social control extends to the actual feeling within. For example, in most human groups, to feel either too much or too little grief is to be subjected to negative sanctions. A person who feels little or no grief over the death of a parent would be considered a moral monster. On the other hand, the widow who mourns too long over the dead spouse will be rebuked. She may be told that she is being "morbid." In instances such as these, it is not merely outward expression which is being controlled but especially and mainly inner feeling. As Arlie Hochschild (1979) has indicated, we expend considerable effort doing "emotion work," that is, struggling either to evoke a feeling that our culture deems appropriate or surpressing a feeling that it deems inappropriate. In modern societies, the bride and bridegroom are expected to feel love for each other, although such an expectation is a comparatively recent event in human history. In all societies in human history, it would appear that social control exerts intense pressure on members to hate its tribal or national enemies, especially in times of conflict or war. Much the same can be said for persons defined as internal enemies, such as minorities and deviants. As I suggest, the extremely strong negative feelings mobilized by acts of deviance, especially moral outrage and indignation, are a centrally important aspect of the social control of deviance.

Like feelings, thoughts and beliefs are aspects of the inner life which seem private, yet like feelings, they are also subject to the action of social control. Before Magellan, anyone who thought that the earth might not be flat would have been considered insane. Similarly, in the 1960s and most of the 1970s, activists who thought that the FBI and CIA were doing what they were actually doing were considered paranoid. The thoughts and beliefs of children are rigorously subject to control. For example, when my oldest child was about 4 years old, he went through a period of nightmares about ghosts and threatening animals that would wake him from sleep. Like any other upstanding member of the tribe, I hastened to assure him that the images he had seen in his sleep were not real. (One incident occurred when I was reassuring him after he had awakened from an animal dream. He pointed to a fold in the bedclothes, asking what it was. I said, ''That's just the sheet.'' Only half awake, he shouted in terror: ''A sheep! A sheep!'') At about the same age, he and I were involved in a protracted struggle over the cleanliness of his hands at mealtime. When I asked him to wash his hands, he would inspect them, then show them to me:

> Son: They are not dirty, they're clean.
> Father: But they may have germs on them.

At this remark, he would again inspect his hands:

> Son: I don't see any germs.
> Father: You can't see them, they're too little.

After considerable time, effort, and emotion, I succeeded in convincing my young son that the dream images he had actually seen were not real and the germs that he had never seen were. I had functioned as an agent of social control over his beliefs about reality. Yet in most societies in human history, the situation would have been reversed. The images in the dream would have been considered real, manifestations of the night-wandering spirits of the dead, and the germs on the hands, unseen and, therefore, unreal. To a large extent, the system of social control in a society constructs reality for its members. As shown in Chapter 3, the social construction of reality is a central issue in the sociological approach to mental disorder.

To review so far: all human groups have a system of social control which shapes all areas of experience—behavior, perception, thought, and feeling. This system operates to obtain conformity: acts which meet normative expectations are positively sanctioned, and acts which violate normative expectations are negatively sanctioned. The system acts through both actual sanctions and through those imagined or assumed. Indeed, the imagined response of others to one's acts is probably fully as important as their real responses in the operation of social control. In becoming adult members of the tribe, children quickly learn to forestall punishment and gain reward from others by rehearsing their acts in their imagination. In order to imagine accurately other's responses, the child learns probable viewpoints of others in the society, at least in part. In this process of socialization, self-control becomes a crucial aspect of social control.

Although social control works relentlessly, both within and without, to shape behavior, perception, thought, and feeling, its actions are not automatic and inevitable. Indeed, in any given situation, there is some uncertainty not only as to whether others will respond with sanctions to a given act, even as to what the relevant expectations are. In real life, the provenance of norms and sanctions is a matter of interpretation and negotiation. In most situations, the police seem to believe and act as if they have considerable discretion in deciding whether or not a crime has been committed. Police may define behavior which could be seen as vandalism as a prank: "Boys will be boys." Furthermore, if they decide that a crime has been committed, they seem to believe and act as if they had considerable discretion to decide whether or not to sanction the purported offender. Relentlessly as it may seem to function when viewed abstractly, in any given situation, the operation of social control has a probabilistic and indeterminate character. This indeterminant character of social control is an essential feature and provides, therefore, considerable matter for deliberation for potential offenders, agents of social control, and for scholars of deviance.

To be sure, one can imagine instances where the ambiguity of the system is vanishingly small. If I seek to remove the gold from Fort Knox by stealth or force of arms, the likelihood that my action, if detected, would not be defined as a violation or not sanctioned negatively may be infinitesmally small. However, it is not inconceivable. For example, it is unlikely, but not impossible, that my action may be defined as an act of national liberation. Needless to say, the odds at this particular moment may be astronomically long. The point is that since the operation of social control involves human beings with the capacity for interpreting and negotiating, there is always an element of uncertainty. To put it in a somewhat different way, each time a shared conformity to expectation is upheld by positive sanctioning or nonconformity is punished, the system of social control is affirmed anew. A social order is stable in so far as it receives continuous affirmation in the lives and actions of its members. At any moment, such affirmation may cease. When it does, the order will change or even disappear. Involvement in a social order requires the continual recreation of that order by its members.

There is an implication of the idea of the indeterminancy of social control which the reader, in his or her capacity as a member of the tribe, may find hard to accept. Crimes and other normative violations are not only relative to the moral order of a particular tribe. The moral order itself is not absolute and fixed but subject to pervasive and continuous testing, in every act, thought, and feeling of its members. Just as the moral order is continually created anew, so every deviant act is a creation, not only of the deviant but of those who interpret his or her behavior as deviant. Categories of deviance are not absolute: There is no such thing as crime per se or, as shown in the chapter on mental illness, psychiatric symptoms per se. The actions that are categorized in this way are selected by each society somewhat differently and in each concrete instance within a given society are interpreted and negotiated anew.

The philosopher Kant said: "Two things fill the mind with awe: the starry sky above and the moral law within." The process of social control, of which the "the moral law within" is a part, is itself an awesome and improbable phenomena. Its operation is usually pervasive, relentless, and invisible, capable of stability for millenia, and equally capable of gradual or instantaneous change. Our discussion now turns to the operation of social control in one particular area, the control of deviance.

THE SOCIETAL REACTION TO DEVIANCE

As already indicated, the concept of *deviance* is widely used in social science to mean violations of normative expectations that are likely to bring responses of indignation and moral outrage from members of the tribe. In this usage, therefore, most normative violations are not seen as instances of deviance. Although belching at a formal dinner would certainly be impolite and would elicit some moral outrage in Western societies, it would not be considered deviant behavior of the level of other violations such as murder, treason, or incest. In Arab societies, however, it is not only polite but expected.

How does one draw the line to distinguish between deviance and other violations? In this discussion, I follow the usage that deviance is a normative violation which may obtain all three of the following responses: moral outrage or stigma, segregation, and labeling. The possibility that these three responses will follow a violation can be used to define deviance.

In this discussion, I argue that stigma is the single most important aspect of the societal reaction to deviance, and that it is also the most intricate. The dimensions of the other two components are straightforward. Segregation implies special procedures for deviants: prisons, asylums, criminal courts, commitment hearings, drunk tanks. All societies have a particular status reserved for deviants and formal procedures for demoting offenders into that status and for promoting them back into the status of normal members of society. We return to this issue in the discussion of status lines.

Labeling, in the sense that it is used here, is one particular aspect of the process of the segregation of deviants into a special status. By virtue of the special procedures of segregation, the offender receives an official label (i.e., thief, convict, schizophrenic, mental patient, prostitute). These labels or status names are also related to stigmatization, however, since they always carry a heavy weight of moral condemnation.

At the core of the societal reaction to deviance is the process of stigmatization. Deviance is that behavior which arouses extraordinarily strong collective loathing. A deviant is that person whose normative violations have aroused strong emotions in the other members of the society. In the process of labeling, this moral opprobrium somehow becomes attached to the deviant; he or she is stigmatized.

In order to understand the societal reaction, it is necessary to realize that the emotional reaction to deviance is usually in excess of the appropriate response. I call this excess, which may be quite small or very large, the *surplus emotional response*. Stigma occurs because of the surplus.

How is it possible to speak of a surplus emotional response? There is a difficult judgment involved, because there is always a component of the emotional response to deviance which is appropriate. A social order is built upon predictable behavior. Unpredictable behavior often brings social transactions to a standstill and therefore gives rise to fear and anger. Consider one of the rules of the road, "Stay on the right side of the road." There is nothing inherently correct about the right side of the road. The left would do equally well, as it does in England. Once chosen, however, it becomes sacrosanct. The social system of the highways does not work perfectly or even very well, since there are many collisions. Nevertheless, driving on the wrong side of the road is a normative violation that brings very strong negative emotions of anger and fear: "You crazy son-of-a-bitch, you're trying to kill me!" The shared expectations of the highway bring some predictability to behavior and therefore a measure of safety.

Oddly enough, the repeated violation of the highway code, even though it may have deadly results, is not highly stigmatized. For reasons which are obscure to me, in this country, the societal reaction to violations of the rules of the road, rather than arousing an excess emotional response, does the opposite. There seems to be a deficit rather than a surplus emotional response. The punishment of traffic violations is notoriously light compared with other kinds of offenses of comparable harm or injury. It is significant that there is no vernacular label, a short and opprobrious epithet, comparable to thief or whore, for the long-term traffic offender.

On the other hand, there are the stigmatized offenses, such as those against person or property, the rules of reality, sobriety, and sexual propriety. There is always a label, both official and vernacular, for these violators and for their violations. These labels are surface manifestation of a deep and intense emotional response involving fear, anger, and / or embarrassment. Why these particular emotions? One reason for fear arousal has already been indicated in the discussion of the rules of the road. Normative behavior gives rise to a predictable world in a very concrete and practical way. Adherence to conventions of speech, dress, and facial expression allows each of us to collaborate with others with a minimum of effort and conflict. Suppose you are walking by yourself in a secluded section of a park in a strange city. If you meet a stranger who is bizarrely dressed, speaks in an odd way, and / or shows a facial expression that seems inappropriate to the context, you would probably be frightened because you would not know what to expect. On the other hand, the same stranger in the same situation, if he is conforming in dress, speech, and facial expression may not be particularly fearful. Every item of dress, word, and fleeting facial expression brings reassurance of predictability.

There is another way in which normative violations generate fear which is somewhat different from the simple issue of the predictability of specific actions. As already indicated, most of the reality of the world that is experienced by human beings is socially constructed. Wholesale violations of social norms shatter this world. In a racist society, any perturbation of the color line may be experienced as cataclysmic. There is a sense of shock, at least initially, even

[margin notes, handwritten: Might/not be / the fear can be / more attributed / to avenge, eg, / danger / anything that / changed, not / custom, not / to ontological / insecurity? / Does driving / on the right itself / connect / to my sense / to my identity?]

when the violations are local and temporary. For me, the first few days of driving on the left side of the road in England has a nightmare quality. Violations of constitutive social norms give rise to ontological fear, that is, the fear that reality itself is collapsing.

The explanation of the emotions of anger and resentment that deviance arouses corresponds to the link between unpredictability and fear previously discussed. Unpredictability gives rise not only to danger but to frustration. It is difficult to get through a social transaction with a person who is breaking the rules. Frustration is the basic context for anger and resentment, particularly where there is even a suspicion that the frustration is intentional. Most members of the tribe, most of the time, suspect that deviance is willed. Anger is the result.

The emotion of embarrassment that arises in connection with deviance is more difficult to explain. Embarrassment usually arises in contexts where a person looses face in public. Humiliation is a very strong form of the same emotion. It is easy to see that the rule-breaker himself would be embarrassed, even if he is the only one who perceives his gaffe, as suggested in the quotation from Bell concerning inappropriate clothing. But what about the others who witness the rule violation? Why should they be embarrassed? The answer to this question is not at all obvious.

It would appear that persons who are cooperating with each other in managing a social transaction necessarily and inevitably identify with each other. Suppose I am involved with another person in lifting a table. In order to smoothly coordinate our actions, I must see, the whole transaction not only from my point of view but from the other persons as well. This kind of identification is not moral and empathic, at least not in the first instance. It is simply practical. To understand the speech of another person, even if I happen to dislike that person with great intensity, I necessarily must take that person's point of view, to locate myself with respect to that person's position, to grasp the meaning of the speech. This kind of process is referred to as *role-taking* and is thought to be the basis of interaction between human beings that is distinctively social. The idea of social norm as an infinite series of shared attributions predicates role-taking.

Given the phenomenon of role-taking, the basis of embarrassment over deviance by on-lookers can be grasped. On-lookers are embarrassed over acts of deviance because they almost automatically identify with other members of the tribe. Perhaps it is for this reason that most people conspire to avoid embarrassing others, generating tact about tact. It is not merely kindness but self-protection. Embarrassment is extremely painful: blushing, averting the gaze, looking at the floor, wishing to escape the scene yet feeling paralyzed and shamed. The pain can be direct for oneself or vicarious for another. The pain of embarrassment is an important aspect of the emotional response to deviance as are the emotions of anger and fear.

At least a part of emotional response to deviance is usually displaced on to the deviants from other areas of the individual's life. Deviants (and enemies and strangers, as well) are heirs to our childhood fears of the boogie man, of the dark, of all that is unknown and menacing. It is this displacement of emotion that gives rise to the indelibility of stigma and to many of the other peculiarities of the societal reaction.

For example, it long has been observed that there is a cycle in the societal reaction to deviance that contains three phases: quiescence, exposé, reform or repression, followed by a repeat of the cycle. (Lemert, 1951: 55–64). Public attention to prisons and mental hospitals is particularly marked by this cycle, but it can also be observed in the cycle of police attention to drunks and vice. This cycle is difficult to understand on rational grounds, since reasonable attempts to solve outstanding social problems would be marked by a more or less constant level of concern and attention. When based on irrational emotions, however, responses are apt to be too little or too much. That is, these emotions are denied until some shocking event necessitates action. When this occurs, there is usually an overreaction, a hysterical outburst of concern. The denial of emotion corresponds to the phase of quiescence; the second phase, the exposé, is the trigger for the last phase, the hysterical overkill of the phase of reform or repression.

The effects of the surplus emotional response to deviance can also be seen in another way. The indelibility of stigma results from the surplus, since it is displaced and therefore quite irrational. The formal structure of retribution or treatment never quite removes all the stigma; the ex-offender or ex-mental patient who has "served his time" or been "cured" still carries some of the stigma of deviance in most cases. The irrational component of stigma also helps explain the cyclical character of the societal reaction. Really effective reform is difficult to mobilize because formally designated deviants are tainted by stigma: their cause is subtly discounted in the political process. A flagrant version of this process can be seen in public reaction to gangland killings: "Let them kill each other off." But it also applies, in a more subtle way, to all societal responses to deviance.

Another example of the discounting process can be seen in some remarks once made to me by a member of the Chamber of Deputies in Italy. This deputy was describing some of the notorious flaws in the mental health system in Italy. When I asked him why there were no reform bills in the Chamber, he said: "No one wants to defend the mentally ill. In Italy they are called '*pozzi*.' If I were to initiate a reform law, my opponents would say that I am *pozzi* too" (at this point he makes a circular motion with his index finger pointed at his temple). The mentally ill are so tainted emotionally that their taint may rub off on their protectors. For this reason, it is difficult to mount a rational program for the management of deviance. Most programs are marked either by impulsive action, on the one hand, or by pretense, on the other, corresponding to the hysterical or to the denial phase in the dynamics of collective emotion.

As can be seen quickly from the preceding discussion, some of the ideas used in outlining the social control of deviance are vague and elusive. It is easy to point to the procedures and labels used in the segregation of formally certified deviants. But where do we find the emotional responses which have been emphasized in this discussion? How can one tell if there is a surplus emotional response or a deficit? Similarly in the discussion of the normative system, one can easily locate and list laws and codes which are part of the formal system. But how can one find the unwritten rules and the unstated codes?

These are important questions, and they are difficult to answer. Investigations of these issues are occurring at the frontier of social science and psychology. A very conservative position to take would be that until there is a wealth of agreed-upon facts about these matters, they should be left out of the reckoning. I take an alternative position. All of us act upon our understanding of emotional responses and unstated rules everyday. This discussion will appeal to the untutored intuition of the reader. To be competent in social interaction, one must be an "expert" in these matters, although one's expertise is so taken for granted that it is hardly ever acknowledged. I believe the conservative position on evidence and fact in social science is a useful strategy for research and teaching, but it is quite incomplete. To rely completely on formal, stated knowledge in social science is to make us foreigners in our own country, having only textbook knowledge of the language and the customs, and therefore really not understanding even the simplest social transaction, let alone the more complex and subtle ones. This book will appeal to both scientific knowledge and to the reader's intuition in order to convey a sophisticated understanding of deviance and social control.

CONCLUSION

In the preceding discussion, the theory of the social control of deviant behavior has been outlined. The theory posits a system for obtaining conforming behavior that is unique to each particular society. The principal components of the system are a vast set of norms which are supported by sanctions. Deviance in a particular system is those normative violations which arouse public outrage and can result in segregation and labeling of the offenders. Finally, the procedures for segregation and labeling result in a status line that divides offenders from nonoffenders. The concept of the *status line* suggests a way of interpreting the causation and management of deviance that is alternative to perspectives that focus on individuals.

What is the advantage of the social control perspective? Is it anything more than a new set of special terms? One advantage has already been suggested in using special terms. Concepts like social control, norms, and deviance help the analyst to disengage from the culture-bound perspective of the society being studied. They are general terms applicable to any society, so that comparisons are made easily. Furthermore, these terms help to detach the argument from the emotional values of a particular society, so that objectivity is increased.

There is a second advantage that has not been mentioned yet in this discussion. The social control perspective is much broader than the individual perspective in that it does not prejudge in conflicts between individual deviants and society. The individual perspective suggests two questions: What causes deviance, and how can it be stopped? These are important questions, but they do not exhaust the kinds of questions that should be asked about deviance. There are historical questions concerning social control: why does a particular society define as deviant a behavior which another society does not? For example, the individual perspective does not exhaust the issue of marijuana use in our era. Why do young people smoke marijuana, and how can it be stopped? A more interesting question is, Who opposes marijuana use, and why is this opposition so strong? Why is marijuana use more severely penalized than the use of alcohol and tranquilizers? The social control perspective calls attention to the system of norms and sanctions as well as to the offenders and their offenses.

One tactic in understanding deviance concerns broad classes of deviance. As suggested in later chapters, crime is produced by criminals, but it is also produced by legislatures. If a legislature were to change the laws governing corporation violations and other ''white-collar'' crimes to criminal, rather than civil, actions, it could create thousands of criminals overnight. A move in the opposite direction is currently happening in psychiatry: it has been agreed that homosexuality is not a mental illness. To the extent that this new definition is accepted by psychiatrists and other key societal agents, thousands of homosexuals will be promoted out of their deviant status.

The social control perspective can also be applied to particular cases of deviance. Why are some offenders detected and punished and others ignored? This is the basic question asked by the ''labeling'' approach to deviance. This approach is concerned with the contingencies that give rise to status demotion for some offenders and not for others. It is also concerned with the effects of segregation, labeling, and stigma on ''chronicity'' (i.e., on the stability of rule-breaking behavior). During one point in English history, a man convicted of theft was branded with an F (for felon) on his forehead. This action insured a career of robbery, since a person so branded could never obtain honest employment. This was an extreme instance of the way in which the societal reaction to deviance produced further deviance. The labeling approach concerns the ways in which society produces deviance, sometimes in ways that are considerably more subtle than branding. Jerome Frank (1961), among others, has addressed this issue as it concerns mental illness:

> By teaching people to regard certain types of distress or behavioral oddities as illnesses rather than as normal reactions to life's stresses, harmless eccentricities, or moral weaknesses, it may cause alarm and increase the demand for psychotherapy. This may explain the curious fact that the use of psychotherapy tends to keep pace with its availability. The greater the number of treatment facilities and the more widely they are known, the larger the number of persons seeking their help. Psychotherapy is the only form of treatment which at least to some extent, appears to create the illness it treats [pp. 6–7].

As is the case with most other areas of human behavior, our understanding of deviance is at a very elementary level. The social control perspective offers the opportunity for broadening the level of analysis and therefore of increasing our awareness in a complex and confusing area of inquiry.

Residual Deviance

3

ONE source of immediate embarrassment to any social theory of "mental illness" is that the terms used in referring to these phenomena in our society prejudge the issue. The medical metaphor "mental illness" suggests a determinate process that occurs within the individual: the unfolding and development of disease. In order to avoid this assumption, we will utilize sociological, rather than medical concepts to formulate the problem. Particularly crucial to the formulation of the problem is the idea of psychiatric "symptoms," which is applied to the behavior that is taken to signify the existence of an underlying mental illness. Since in the great majority of cases of mental illness, the existence of this underlying illness is unproved, we need to discuss "symptomatic" behavior in terms that do not involve the assumption of illness.

Two concepts seem to be suited best to the task of discussing psychiatric symptoms from a sociological point of view: *rule-breaking* and *deviance*. Rule-breaking refers to behavior that is in clear violation of the agreed-upon rules of the group. These rules are usually discussed by sociologists as social norms. If the symptoms of mental illness are to be construed as violations of social norms, it is necessary to specify the type of norms involved. Most norm violations do not cause the violator to be labeled as mentally ill, but as ill-mannered, ignorant, sinful, criminal, or perhaps just harried, depending on the type of norm involved. There are innumerable norms, however, over which consensus is so complete that the members of a group appear to take them for granted. A host of such norms surround even the simplest conversation: a person engaged in conversation is expected to face toward his partner, rather than directly away from him; if his gaze is toward the partner, he is expected to look toward the other's eyes, rather than, say, toward his forehead; to stand at a proper conversational distance, neither one inch away nor across the room, and so on. A person who regularly violated these expectations probably would not be thought to be merely ill-bred, but as strange, bizarre, and frightening, because his behavior violates the assumptive world of the group, the world that is construed to be the only one that is natural, decent, and possible.

The concept of deviance used here will follow Becker's (1963) usage. He argues that deviance can be most usefully considered as a quality of people's response to an act, rather than as a characteristic of the act itself.

> Social groups create deviance by making the rules whose infraction constitutes deviance, and by applying those rules to *particular people* and labeling them as outsiders . . . deviance is not a quality of the act the person commits, but rather a consequence of the application by others of rules and sanctions to an "offender." *The deviant is one to whom that label has successfully been applied;* deviant behavior is behavior that people so label [p. 9; italics rearranged.]

By this definition, deviants are not a group of people who have committed the same act, but are a group of people who have been stigmatized as deviants.

Becker argues that the distinction between rule-breaking and deviance is necessary for scientific purposes:

> Since deviance is, among other things, a consequence of the responses of others to a person's act, students of deviance cannot assume that they are dealing with a homogeneous category when they study people who have been labeled deviant. That is, they cannot assume that these people have actually . . . broken some rule, because the process of labeling may not be infallible. . . . Furthermore, they cannot assume that the category of those labeled deviant will contain all those who actually have broken a rule, for many offenders may escape apprehension and thus fail to be included in the population of "deviants" they study. Insofar as the category lacks homogeneity and fails to include all the cases that belong in it, one cannot reasonably expect to find common factors of personality or life situation that will account for the supposed deviance [p. 9].

For the purpose of this discussion, we will conform to Becker's separation of rule-breaking and deviance. Rule-breaking will refer to a class of acts, violations of social norms, and deviance to particular acts which have been publicly and officially labeled as norm violations.

Using Becker's distinction, we can categorize most psychiatric symptoms as instances of residual rule-breaking or residual deviance. The culture of the group provides a vocabulary of terms for categorizing many norm violations: crime, perversion, drunkenness, and bad manners are familiar examples. Each of these terms is derived from the type of norm broken and, ultimately, from the type of behavior involved. After exhausting these categories, however, there is always a residue of the most diverse kinds of violations for which the culture provides no explicit label. For example, although there is great cultural variation in what is defined as decent or real, each culture tends to reify its definition of decency and reality and so provides no way of handling violations of its expectations in these areas. The typical norm governing decency or reality, therefore, literally "goes without saying," and its violation is unthinkable for most of its members. For the convenience of the society in construing those instances of unnamable rule-breaking which are called to its attention, these violations may be lumped together into a residual category: witchcraft, spirit possession, or, in our own society, mental illness. In this discussion, the diverse kinds of rule-breaking for which our society provides no explicit label and which, therefore, sometimes lead to the labeling of the violator as mentally ill, will be considered to be technically *residual rule-breaking*.

Let us consider further some of the implications of a definition of psychiatric "symptoms" as instances of residual deviance. In *Behavior in Public Places*, Goffman (1964) develops the idea that there is a complex of social norms that regulate the way in which a person may behave when in the presence, or potentially in the presence, of other persons. Goffman's discussion of the norms regarding "involvement," particularly, illustrates how such psychiatric symptoms as withdrawal and hallucinations may be regarded as violations of residual rules.

Noting that lolling and loitering are usually specifically prohibited in codes of law, Goffman goes on to point out that there is a much more elaborate set of norms centering around the expectation that a person appearing in public should be involved or engaged in doing something:

> The rule against "having no purpose," or being disengaged, is evident in the exploitation of untaxing involvements to rationalize or mask desired lolling—a way of covering one's physical presence in a situation with a veneer of acceptable visible activity. Thus when individuals want a "break" in their work routine, they may remove themselves to a place where it is acceptable to smoke and there smoke in a pointed fashion. Certain minimal "recreational" activities are also used as covers for disengagement, as in the case of "fishing" off river banks where it is guaranteed that no fish will disturb one's reverie, or "getting a tan" on the beach—activity that shields reverie or sleep, although, as with hoboes' lolling, a special uniform may have to be worn, which proclaims and institutionalizes the relative inactivity. As might be expected, when the context firmly provides a dominant involvement that is outside the situation, as when riding in a train or airplane, then gazing out the window, or reverie, or sleeping may be quite permissible. In short, the more the setting guarantees that the participant has not withdrawn from what he ought to be involved in, the more liberty it seems he will have to manifest what would otherwise be considered withdrawal in the situation [1964:58–59].

The rule requiring that an adult be "involved" when in public view is unstated in our society, yet so taken for granted that individuals almost automatically shield their lack of involvement in socially acceptable ways, as illustrated in the quotation. Thus the rule of involvement would seem to be a residual rule.

Two types of involvements that Goffman discusses are particularly relevant to a discussion of residual deviance: "away" and "occult involvements." "Away" is described in this manner:

> While outwardly participating in an activity within a social situation, an individual can allow his attention to turn from what he and everyone else considered the real or serious world, and

give himself up for a time to a playlike world in which he alone participates. This kind of inward emigration from the gathering may be called "away," and we find that strict regulations obtain regarding it.

Perhaps the most important kind of away is that through which the individual relives some past experiences or rehearses some future ones, this taking the form of what is variously called reverie, brown study, woolgathering, daydreaming or autistic thinking. At such times the individual may demonstrate his absence from the current situation by a preoccupied, faraway look in his eyes, or by a sleeplike stillness of his limbs, or by that special class of side involvements that can be sustained in an utterly "unconscious" abstracted manner—humming, doodling, drumming the fingers on a table, hair twisting, nose picking, scratching [1964:69–70].

This discussion is relevant to the psychiatric symptoms which come under the rubric of "withdrawal," showing that the behavior which is called "withdrawal" in itself is not socially unacceptable. An "away" is met with public censure only when it occurs in a socially unacceptable context. But this is to say that there are residual rules governing the context in which "aways" may take place. When an "away" violates these rules, it is apt to be called "withdrawal" and taken as evidence of mental illness.

"Occult involvement" is defined as a subtype of "awayness":

There is a kind of awareness where the individual gives others the impression, whether warranted or not, that he is not aware that he is "away." This is the area of what psychiatry terms "hallucinations" and delusionary states. Corresponding to these "unnatural" verbal activities, there are unnatural bodily ones, where the individual's activity is patiently tasklike but not "understandable" or "meaningful." The unnatural action may even involve the holding or grasping of something, as when an adult mental patient retains a tight hold on a doll or a fetish-like piece of cloth. Here the terms "mannerism," "ritual act," or "posturing" are applied, which, like the term "unnatural," are clear enough in their way but hardly tell us with any specificity what it is that characterizes "natural" acts [1964:75–76].

At first glance, it would seem that if there were ever a type of behavior that in itself would be seen as abnormal, it would be "occult involvements." As Goffman notes, however, there is an element of cultural definition even with "occult involvements": "There are societies in which conversation with a spirit not present is as acceptable when sustained by properly authorized persons as is conversation over a telephone in American society [1964:79]." Furthermore, he points out that even in American society, there are occasions in which "occult involvement" is not censured: "Those who attend a seance would not consider it inappropriate for the medium to interact with "someone on the other side," whether they believe this to be staged or a genuine interaction. And certainly we define praying as acceptable when done at proper occasions [1964:79]." Thus, talking to spirits or praying to God are not improper in themselves; indeed, they are seen as legitimate modes of activity when they follow the proprieties—that is, when they occur in the socially proper circumstances and are conducted by persons recognized as legitimately, even though occultly, involved.

Two significant implications follow from this discussion of the etiquette of involvement. The first is that such psychiatric symptoms as withdrawal, hallucinations, continual muttering, posturing, etc., may be categorized as violations of certain social norms—those norms that are so taken for granted that they are not explicitly verbalized, which we have called residual rules. In particular instances discussed here, the residual rule concerned involvement in public places. It is true, of course, that various specific aspects of the involvement rule occasionally are found, for example, in books of etiquette. Here for example, is a typical proscription concerning involvement with one's own person in public places: .

> Men should never look in the mirror nor comb their hair in public. At most a man may straighten his necktie and smooth his hair with his hand. It is probably unnecessary to add that it is most unattractive to scratch one's head, to rub one's face or touch one's teeth, or to clean one's fingernails in public. All these things should be done privately [Fenwick, 1948:11; quoted in Goffman, 1964].

Although many such informal rules could be pointed to, it is important to note that they are all situationally specific. There is nowhere codified a general principle of involvement or even self-involvement. Unlike codified principles, such as the Ten Commandments, it is one of those expectations that it is felt should govern the behavior of every decent person, even though it goes unsaid. Because it goes unsaid, we are not equipped by our culture to smoothly categorize violations of such a rule but rather may resort to a residual catch-all category of violations (i.e., symptoms of mental illness).

If it proves to be correct that most symptoms of mental illness can be systematically classified as violations of culturally particular normative networks, then these symptoms may be removed from the realm of universal physical events, where they now tend to be placed by psychiatric theory, along with other culture-free symptoms such as fever, and be investigated sociologically and anthropologically like any other item of social behavior.

A second implication of the redefinition of psychiatric symptoms as residual deviance is the great emphasis that this perspective puts on the context in which the "symptomatic" behavior occurs. As Goffman repeatedly shows, "aways," "occult involvements," and other kinds of rule violations do not in themselves bring forth censure; it is only when socially unqualified persons perform these acts or perform them in inappropriate contexts. That is, these acts are objectionable when they occur in a manner that does not conform to the unstated, but nevertheless operative, etiquette that governs them. Although recently psychiatric discussions of symptomatology have begun to display considerable interest in the social context, it is still true that psychiatric diagnosis tends to focus on the pattern of symptomatic behavior itself, to the neglect of the context in which the symptom occurs. The significance of this tendency in psychiatric diagnostic procedures is discussed later.[1] The remainder of this chapter is devoted to a

---

[1]See Chapter 6 on the relationship between symptoms, context, and meaning.

discussion of the origins, prevalence, and course of the behavior that we have defined here as residual rule-breaking.

THE ORIGINS OF RESIDUAL RULE-BREAKING

It is customary in psychiatric research to seek a single generic source or at best a small number of sources for mental illness. The redefinition of psychiatric symptoms as residual deviance immediately suggests, however, that there should be an unlimited number of sources of deviance. The first proposition follows.

Proposition 1: _Residual rule-breaking arises from fundamentally diverse sources_. Four distinct types of sources are discussed here: organic, psychological, external stress, and volitional acts of innovation or defiance. The organic and psychological origins of residual rule-breaking are widely noted and are not discussed at length here. It has been demonstrated repeatedly that particular cases of mental disorder had their origin in genetic, biochemical, or physiological conditions. Psychological sources are also frequently indicated: peculiarity of up-bringing and training have been reported often, particularly in the psychoanalytic literature. The great majority of precise and systematic studies of causation of mental disorder have been limited to either organic or psychological sources.

It is widely granted, however, that psychiatric symptoms can also arise from external stress: from drug ingestion, the sustained fear and hardship of combat, and from deprivation of food, sleep, and even sensory experience. Excerpts from reports on the consequences of stress will illustrate the rule-breaking behavior that is generated by this less familiar source.

Physicians have long known that toxic substances can cause psychotic-like symptoms when ingested in appropriate doses. Recently a wide variety of substances have been the subject of experimentation in producing "model psychoses." Drugs such as a mescaline and LSD-25, particularly, have been described as producing fairly close replicas of psychiatric symptoms, such as visual hallucinations, loss of orientation to space and time, interference with thought processes, etc. Here is an excerpt from a report by a qualified psychologist who had taken LSD-25:

> One concomitant of LSD that I shared with other subjects was distortion of the time sense. The subjective clock appeared to race. This was observed even at 25 milligrams in counting 60 seconds. My tapping rate was also speeded up. On the larger dose (½ gram) my time sense was dipslaced by hours. I thought the afternoon was well spent when it was only 1:00 P.M. I could look at my watch and realize the error, but I continued to be disoriented in time. The time sense depends on the way time is "filled," and I was probably responding to the quickened tempo of experience.
>
> This was in fact, my overwhelming impression of LSD. Beginning with the physiological sensations (lightheadedness, excitement) I was shortly flooded by a montage of ideas, images, and feelings that seemed to thrust themselves upon me unbidden. I had glimpses of very bright thoughts, like a fleeting insight into the psychotic process, which I wanted to write down. . . . But they pushed each other aside. Once gone, they could not be recaptured because the parade of new images could not be stopped [C. C. Bennett, 1960:606–607].

The time disorientation described is a familiar psychiatric symptom, as is the ideational "pressure," which is usually described as a feature of manic excitement.

Combat psychosis and psychiatric symptoms arising from starvation have been repeatedly described in the psychiatric literature. Psychotic symptoms resulting from sleeplessness are less familiar. One instance is used to illustrate this reaction. Brauchi and West (1959:11) reported the symptoms of two participants in a radio marathon that required them to talk alternately every 30 minutes. After 168 hours, one of the contestants felt that he and his opponent belonged to a secret club of nonsleepers. He accused his girl-friend of kissing an observer, even though she was with him at the time. He felt he was being punished, had transient auditory and visual hallucinations, and became suggestible, he and his opponent exhibiting a period of *folie à deux* when the delusions and hallucinations of the one were accepted by the other. He showed persistence of his psychotic symptoms, with delusions about secret agents, and felt that he was responsible for the Israeli–Egyptian conflict. His reactions contain many elements that psychiatrists would describe as paranoid and depressive features.

There have been a number of recent studies which show that deprivation of sensory stimulation can cause hallucinations and other symptoms. In one such study, Heron (1961) reported on subjects who were cut off from sensations:

> Male college students were paid to lie 24 hours a day on a comfortable bed in a lighted semi-soundproof cubicle . . . wearing translucent goggles which admitted diffuse light but prevented pattern vision. Except when eating or at toilet, they wore cotton gloves and cardboard cuffs . . . in order to limit tactile perceptions [p. 8].

The subjects stayed from 2 to 3 days. Twenty-five of the 29 subjects reported hallucinations, which usually were initially simple and became progressively more complex over time. Three of the subjects believed their visions to be real:

> One man thought that he saw things coming at him and showed head withdrawal quite consistently when this happened; a second was convinced that we were projecting pictures on his goggles by some sort of movie camera; a third felt that someone else was in the cubicle with him [p. 17].

Merely monotonous environments, as in long-distance driving or flying, are now thought to be capable of generating symptoms. The following excerpt is taken from a series on psychiatric symptoms in military aviation.

> A pilot was flying a bomber at 40,000 feet and had been continuing straight and level for about an hour. There was a haze over the ground which prevented a proper view and rendered the horizon indistinct. The other member of the crew was sitting in a separate place out of the pilot's view, and the two men did not talk to each other. Suddenly the pilot felt detached from his surroundings and then had the strong impression that the aircraft had one wing down and was turning. Without consulting his instruments he corrected the attitude, but the aircraft went to a spiral dive because it had in fact been flying straight and level. The pilot was very lucky to

recover from the spiral dive, and when he landed the airframe was found to be distorted [from the stress caused by the dive].

On examining the pilot, no psychiatric abnormality was found. . . . As the man had no wish to give up flying and was in fact physically and mentally fit, he was offered an explanation of the phenomenon and was reassured. He returned to flying duties [A.M.H. Bennett, 1961:166]

In this case, the symptoms (depersonalization and spatial disorientation), occurring as they did in a real-life situation, could easily have resulted in a fatal accident. In laboratory studies of model psychoses, the consequences are usually easily controlled. Particularly relevant to this discussion is the role of reassurance of the subject by the experimenter, after the experiment is over.

In all of the laboratory studies (as in this last case as well), the persons who have had "psychotic" experiences are reassured; they are told, for example, that the experiences they had were solely due to the situation that they were placed in, and that anyone else placed in such a situation would experience similar sensations. In other words, the implications of the rule-breaking for the rule-breaker's social status and self-conception are "normalized." Suppose, however, for purposes of argument, that a diabolical experiment were performed in which subjects, after having exhibited the psychotic symptoms under stress, were "labeled." That is, they were told that the symptoms were not a normal reaction, but a reliable indication of deep-seated psychological disorder in their personality. Suppose, in fact, that such labeling were continued in their ordinary lives. Would such a labeling process stablize rule-breaking which would have otherwise been transitory? This question is considered under Proposition 3, following, and in Chapter 4.

Returning to the consideration of origins, rule-breaking finally can be seen as a volitional act of innovation or rebellion. Two examples from art history illustrate the deliberate breaking of residual rules. It is reported that the early reactions of the critics and the public to the paintings of the French impressionists were ones of disbelief and dismay; the colors, particularly, were thought to be so unreal as to be evidence of madness. It is ironic that in the ensuing struggle, the Impressionists and their followers effected some changes in the color norms of the public. Today, we accept the colors of the Impressionists (as in Pepsi-Cola ads) without a second glance.

The Dada movement provides an example of an art movement deliberately conceived to violate, and thereby reject, existing standards of taste and value. The jewel-encrusted book of Dada, which was to contain the greatest treasures of contemporary civilization, was found to be filled with toilet-paper, grass, and similar materials. A typical *objet d'art* produced by Dadaism was a fur-lined teacup. A climactic event in the movement was the Dada Exposition given at the Berlin Opera House. All of the celebrities of the German art world and dignitaries of the Weimar Republic were invited to attend the opening night. The first item of the evening was a poetry-reading contest, in which there were fourteen contestants. Since the fourteen read their poems simultaneously, the evening soon ended in a riot.

The examples of residual rule-breaking given here are not presented as scientifically impeccable instances of this type of behavior. There are many problems connected with reliability in these areas, particularly with the material on behavior resulting from drug ingestion and sleep and sensory deprivation. Much of this material is simply clinical or autobiographical impressions of single, isolated instances. In the studies that have been conducted, insufficient attention is usually paid to research design, systematic techniques of data collection, and devices to guard against experimenter or subject bias.

Of the many questions of a more general nature that are posed by these examples, one of the more interesting is: are the "model psychoses" produced by drugs or food, sleep, or sensory deprivation actually identical to "natural" psychoses, or, on the other hand, are the similarities only superficial, masking fundamental differences between the laboratory and the natural rule-breaking? The opinions of researchers are split on this issue. Many investigators state that model and real psychoses are basically the same. According to a recent report, in the autobiographical, clinical, and experimental accounts of sensory deprivation, Bleuler's cardinal symptoms of schizophrenia frequently appear: disturbances of associations, disharmony of affect, autism, ambivalence, disruption of secondary thought processes accompanied by regression to primary processes, impairment of reality-testing capacity, distortion of body image, depersonalization, delusions, and hallucinations (Rosenzwerg, 1959:326). Other researchers, however, insist that there are fundamental differences between experimental and genuine psychoses.

The controversy over model psychoses provides evidence of a basic difficulty in the scientific study of mental disorder. Although there is an enormous literature on the description of psychiatric symptoms, at this writing, scientifically respectable descriptions of the major psychiatric symptoms, that is to say, descriptions which have been shown to be precise, reliable, and valid, do not exist (Scott, 1958:29–45). It is not only that studies which demonstrate the precision, reliability, and validity of measures of symptomatic behavior have not been made, but that the very basis of such studies, operational definitions of psychiatric symptoms, have yet to be formulated. In physical medicine, there are instruments that yield easily verified, repeatable measures of disease symptoms; the thermometer used in detecting the presence of fever is an obvious example. The analogous instruments in psychiatric medicine, questionnaires, behavior rating scales, etc. which yield verifiable measures of the presence of some symptom pattern (e.g., paranoid ideation) have yet to be found, tested, and agreed upon.

In the absence of scientifically acceptable evidence, we can only rely on our own assessment of the evidence in conjunction with our appraisal of the conflicting opinions of the psychiatric investigators. In this case, there is at present no conclusive answer, but the weight of evidence seems to be that there is some likelihood that the model psychoses are not basically dissimilar to ordinary psychoses. Therefore, it appears that the first proposition, that there are many diverse sources of residual rule-breaking, is supported by available knowledge.

PREVALENCE

The second proposition concerns the prevalence of residual rule-breaking in entire and ostensibly normal populations. This prevalence is roughly analogous to what medical epidemiologists call the "total" or "true" prevalence of mental symptoms.

Proposition 2: *Relative to the rate of treated mental illness, the rate of unrecorded residual rule-breaking is extremely high.* There is evidence that gross violations of rules are often not noticed or, if noticed, rationalized as eccentricity. Apparently, many persons who are extremely withdrawn or who "fly off the handle" for extended periods of time, who imagine fantastic events, or who hear voices or see visions, are not labeled as insane either by themselves or others.[2] Their rule-breaking, rather, is unrecognized, ignored, or rationalized. This pattern of inattention and rationalization is called "normalization."[3]

In addition to the kind of evidence just cited, there are a number of epidemiological studies of total prevalence. There are numerous problems in interpreting the results of these studies; the major difficulty is that the definition of mental disorder is different in each study, as are the methods used to screen cases. These studies represent, however, the best available information and can be used to estimate total prevalence.

A convenient summary of findings is presented in Plunket and Gordon (1960). These authors compare the methods and populations used in eleven field studies and list rates of total prevalence (in percentage) as 1.7, 3.6, 4.5, 4.7, 5.3, 6.1, 10.9, 13.8, 23.2, 23.3, and 33.3.

Since the Plunkett and Gordon review was published, two elaborate studies of symptom prevalence have appeared, one in Manhattan, the other in Nova Scotia (Srole *et al.*, 1962 and Leighton *et al.*, 1963). In the Midtown Manhattan study, it is reported that 80% of the sample currently had at least one psychiatric symptom. Probably more comparable to the earlier studies is their rating of "impaired because of psychiatric illness," which was applied to 23.4% of the population. In the Stirling County studies, the estimate of current prevalence is 57%, with 20% classified as "Psychiatric Disorder with Significant Impairment."

How do these total rates compare with the rates of treated mental disorder? One of the studies cited by Plunkett and Gordon, the Baltimore study reported by Pasamanick (1961:151–155), is useful in this regard since it includes both treated and untreated rates. As compared with the untreated rate of 10.9%, the rate of treatment in state, VA, and private hospitals of Baltimore residents was 0.5% (Pasamanick, 1961:153). That is, for every mental patient there were approximately 20 untreated persons located by the survey. It is possible that the treated rate is too low, however, since patients treated by private physicians were not

---

[2]See, for example, Clausen and Yarrow (1955); Hollingshead and Redlich (1958:172–176); E. Cumming and J. Cumming (1957:92–103).

[3]The term *denial* is used in the same sense as in Cumming and Cumming (1957: Chapter 7).

included. Judging from another study, the New Haven study of treated prevalence, the number of patients treated in private practice is small in comparison with those hospitalized: over 70% of the patients located in that study were hospitalized even though extensive case-finding techniques were employed. The overall treated prevalence in the New Haven study was reported as 0.8%, a figure that is in good agreement with my estimate of 0.7% for the Baltimore study (Hollingshead and Redlich, 1958:199). If we accept 0.8% as an estimate of the upper limit of treated prevalence for the Pasamanick study, the ratio of treated to untreated patients is 1:14. That is, for every patient we should expect to find 14 untreated cases in the community.

One interpretation of this finding is that the untreated patients in the community represent those with less severe disorders, while patients with severe impairments all fall into the treated group. Some of the findings in the Pasamanick study point in this direction. Of the untreated patients, about half are classified as psychoneurotic. Of the psychoneurotics, in turn, about half again are classified as suffering from minimal impairment. At least a fourth of the untreated group, then, involved very mild disorders (Pasamanick, 1961:153–154).

The evidence from the group diagnosed as psychotic does not support this interpretation, however. Almost all of the persons diagnosed as psychotic were judged to have severe impairment; yet half of the diagnoses of psychosis occurred in the untreated group. In other words, according to this study, there were as many untreated as treated cases of psychoses (Pasamanick, 1961:153–154).

In the Manhattan study, a direct comparison by age group was made between the most deviant group (those classified as "incapacitated") and persons actually receiving psychiatric treatment. The results for the groups of younger age (20–40 years) is similar to that in the Pasamanick study: Treated prevalence is roughly 0.6%, and the proportion classified as "incapacitated" is about 1.5%. In the older age group, however, the ratio of treated to treatable changes abruptly. The treated prevalence is about 0.5%, but 4% are designated as "incapacitated" in the population. In the older group, therefore, the ratio of treatable to treated (Srole, 1962) is about 8:1.

Once again, because of lack of complete comparability between studies, conflicting results, and inadequate research designs, the evidence regarding prevalence is not conclusive. The existing weight of evidence appears, however, very strongly to support Proposition 2.

THE DURATION AND CONSEQUENCES
OF RESIDUAL RULE-BREAKING

In most epidemiological research, it is frequently assumed that treated prevalence is an excellent index of total prevalence. The community studies previously discussed, however, suggest that the majority of cases of "mental illness" never receive medical attention. This finding has great significance for a crucial question about residual deviance: given a typical instance of residual rule-breaking, what is its expected course and consequences? Or, to put the same question in medical language, what is the prognosis for a case in which psychiatric signs and symptoms are evident?

The usual working hypothesis for physicians confronted with a sign or symptom is that of progressive development as the inner logic of disease unfolds. The medical framework thus leads one to expect that unless medical intervention occurs, the signs and symptoms of disease are usually harbingers of further, and more serious, consequences for the individual showing the symptoms. This is not to say, of course, that physicians think of all symptoms as being parts of a progressive disease pattern; witness the concept of the "benign" condition. The point is that the imagery that the medical model calls up tends to predispose the physician toward expecting that symptoms are but initial signs of further illness.

The finding that the great majority of persons displaying psychiatric symptoms go untreated leads to the third proposition.

Proposition 3: *Most residual rule-breaking is normalized and is of transitory significance.* The enormously high rates of total prevalence suggest that most residual rule-breaking is unrecognized or rationalized away. For this type of rule-breaking, which is amorphous and uncrystallized, Lemert used the term *primary deviation* (Lemert, 1951: chapter 4). Balint (1957:18) describes similar behavior as "the unorganized phase of illness." Although Balint assumes that patients in this phase ultimately "settle down" to an "organized illness," other outcomes are possible. A person in this stage may "organize" his deviance in other than illness terms (e.g., as eccentricity or genius), or the rule-breaking may terminate when situational stress is removed.

The experience of battlefield psychiatrists can be interpreted to support the hypothesis that residual rule-breaking is usually transitory. Glass (1953) reports that combat neurosis is often self-terminating if the soldier is kept with his unit and given only the most superficial medical attention.[4] Descriptions of child behavior can be interpreted in the same way. According to these reports, most children go through periods in whch at least several of the following kinds of rule-breaking may occur: temper tantrums, head banging, scratching, pinching, biting, fantasy playmates or pets, illusory physical complaints, and fears of sounds, shapes, colors, persons, animals, darkness, weather, ghosts, and so on (Ilg and Ames, 1960:138–188). In the vast majority of instances, however, these behavior patterns do not become stable.

There are, of course, conditions which do fit the model of a progressively unfolding disease. In the case of a patient exhibiting psychiatric symptoms because of general paresis, the early signs and symptoms appear to be good, though not perfect, indicators of later more serious deterioration of both physical health and social behavior. Conditions that have been demonstrated to be of this type are relatively rare, however. Paresis, which was once a major category of

---

[4]Cf. Kardiner and Spiegal (1947: Chapters 3–4).

mental disease, accounts today for only a very minor proportion of mental patients under treatment. Proposition 3 would appear to fit the great majority of mental patients, in whom external stress such as family conflict, fatigue, drugs, and similar factors are often encountered.

Of the first three propositions, the last is both the most crucial for the theory as a whole and the least well supported by existing evidence. It is not a matter of there being great amounts of negative evidence, showing that psychiatric symptoms are reliable indicators of subsequent disease, but that there is little evidence of any kind concerning development of symptoms over time. There are a number of analogies in the history of physical medicine, however, that are suggestive. For example, until the late 1940s, histoplasmosis was thought to be a rare tropical disease with a uniformly fatal outcome (Schwartz and Baum, 1957). Recently, however, it has been discovered that it is widely prevalent and with fatal outcome or even impairment extremely unusual. It is conceivable that most "mental illnesses" may prove to follow the same pattern when adequate longitudinal studies of cases in normal populations have been made.

If residual rule-breaking is highly prevalent among ostensibly "normal" persons and is usually transitory, as suggested by the last two propositions, what accounts for the small percentage of residual rule-breakers who go on to deviant careers? To put the question another way, under what conditions is residual rule-breaking stabilized? The conventional hypothesis is that the answer lies in the rule-breaker himself. The hypothesis suggested here is that the most important single factor (but not the only factor) in the stabilization of residual rule-breaking is the societal reaction. Residual rule-breaking may be stabilized if it is defined to be evidence of mental illness and / or the rule-breaker is placed in a deviant status and begins to play the role of the mentally ill. In order to avoid the implication that mental disorder is merely role-playing and pretense, it is necessary to discuss the social institution of insanity in the next chapter.

The Social Institution
of Insanity

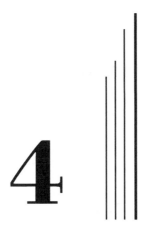

Among psychiatrists, Szasz has been the most outspoken critic of the use of the medical model when applied to "mental illness." His criticism has taken the form that mental illness is a myth that serves functions that are largely nonmedical in nature:

> Our adversaries are not demons, witches, fate, or mental illness. We have no enemy whom we can fight, exorcise, or dispel by "cure." What we do have are *problems in living*—whether these be biologic, economic, political, or sociopsychological. . . . The field to which modern psychiatry addresses itself is vast, and I made no effort to encompass it all. My argument was limited to the proposition that mental illness is a myth, whose function it is to disguise and thus render more palatable the bitter pill of moral conflicts in human relations [1960].

Szasz's formulations of the social, nonmedical functions that the idea of mental illness is made to serve are clear, cogent, and convincing. His conceptualization of the behavior which is symptomatic of "mental illness," however, is open to criticisms of a social–psychological nature.

In the *Myth of Mental Illness* (1960) Szasz proposes that mental disorder be viewed within the framework of "the game-playing model of human behavior [p. 113–1180]." He then describes hysteria, schizophrenia, and other mental disorders as the "impersonation" of sick persons by those whose "real" problem concerns "problems of living." Although Szasz states that role-playing by mental patients may not be completely or even mostly voluntary, the implication is that mental disorder be viewed as a strategy chosen by the individual as a way of obtaining help from others. Thus, the term *impersonation* suggests calculated and deliberate shamming by the patient. Although he notes differences between behavior patterns of hysteria, malingering, and cheating, he suggests that these differences may be mostly a matter of whose point of view is taken in describing the behavior.

INDIVIDUAL AND INTERPERSONAL SYSTEMS IN ROLE-PLAYING

The present discussion also uses the role-playing model to analyze mental disorder but places more emphasis on the involuntary aspects of role-playing than Szasz, who tends to treat role-playing as an individual system of behavior. In many social–psychological discussions, however, role-playing is considered as a part of a social system. The individual plays his role by articulating his behavior with the cues and actions of other persons involved in the transaction. The proper performance of a role is dependent on having a cooperative audience. The proposition may also be reversed: Having an audience that acts toward the individual in a uniform way may lead the actor to play the expected role even if he is not particularly interested in doing so. The "baby of the family" may come to find this role obnoxious, but the uniform pattern of cues and actions that confronts him in the family may lock in with his own vocabulary of responses so that it is inconvenient and difficult for him not to play the part expected of him. To the degree that alternative roles are closed off, the proffered role may come to be the only way the individual can cope with the situation.

One of Szasz' very apt formulations touches upon the social–systemic aspects of role-playing. Szasz (1960) draws an analogy between the role of the mentally ill and the "type-casting" of actors.[1] Some actors get a reputation for playing one type of role, and find it difficult to obtain other roles. Although they may be displeased, they may also come to incorporate aspects of the type-cast role into their self-conceptions and ultimately into their behavior. Findings in several social–psychological studies (Blau, 1956; Benjamins, 1950; Ellis, 1945; Lieberman, 1956) suggest that an individual's role behavior may be shaped by the kinds of "deference" that he regularly receives from others.[2]

One aspect of the voluntariness of role-playing is the extent to which the actor believes in the part he is playing. Although a role may be played cynically, with no belief, or completely sincerely, with whole-hearted belief, many roles are played on the basis of an intricate mixture of belief and disbelief. During the course of a study of a large public mental hospital, several patients told the author in confidence about their cynical use of their symptoms—to frighten new personnel, to escape from unpleasant work details, and so on. Yet, at other times, these *same* patients appear to have been sincere in their symptomatic behavior. Apparently, it was sometimes difficult for them to tell whether they

---

[1]For a discussion of type-casting, see Klapp (1962:5–8 *et passim*).

[2]For a review of experimental evidence, see Mann (1956). For an interesting demonstration of the interrelations between symptoms of patients on the same ward, see Kellam and Chassan (1962).

were playing the role or the role was playing them. Certain types of symp-tomatology are quite interesting in this connection. In cases of patients simulat-ing previous psychotic states and in the behavior pattern known to psychiatrists as the Ganser syndrome, it is apparently almost impossible for the observer to separate feigning of symptoms from involuntary acts with any degree of cer-tainty.

The following case history excerpt from Sadow and Suslick (1961) will illus-trate what psychiatrists have called simulation of a previous psychotic state:

> A 32-year-old white man, an engineer, was readmitted to the hospital because of the recurrence of psychotic behavior. He had been hospitalized twice previously. The first time he had had electroshock treatment and had a remission for 4 years. One of us . . . saw him during his second hospitalization. At that time he was severely regressed, hallucinating freely, had magical and delusional behavior and many ideas of a Messianic nature. He made a good functional recovery after several months of intensive psychotherapy by his private psychiatrist, supplemented with insulin coma treatment. Several years later he had a recurrence of symp-toms and, because of my acquaintance with him during the previous hospitalization, he was referred by his previous therapist. On admission his behavior was bizarre enough to warrant sending him to the disturbed unit. There he immediately took over the unit claiming seniority rights because of his previous stay. When seen he was jovially patronizing, referred to his voices in a smiling manner and interspersed the interview with vague magical inferences of seemingly great significance. He continually made a particular gesture, that of a clock with the hands at the 6 o'clock position. This gesture had been the subject of much inquiry and work on his previous admission. As a result of the prior contact, it was possible to be more direct and enquiring with him than if he had been a new patient. At this point he gave no indications as to the precipitating stimulus of disruptive conflict. During some bantering in which he referred to his current hospitalization as a vacation, or a return of the old grad to his Alma Mater, he was told that this might prove to be an expensive class reunion. (This was in reference to one of his ostensible reasons for discontinuing psychotherapy following his previous disorder, namely, that treatment was too costly.) With almost dramatic swiftness following this remark, his bizarre behavior stopped and be became quite depressed although still communicative. The following day it was possible to transfer him to a less controlled unit and he described in a completely coherent fashion with intense but appropriate emotion that he was extremely angry with his wife for nagging and belittling him. He was afraid he would not be able to control himself and felt that if he were sick like the last time he could avoid a feared outburst of physical violence by being hospitalized. In a few days he was able to recognize that much of the rage at his wife was directed at her current pregnancy. Although a moderate depression persisted, there was no recurrence of the bizarre behavior or the apparent hallucinations. He left the hospital after 3 weeks and returned directly to his job and home [p. 452–458].

What makes "simulation" particularly relevant to a social–systemic theory of mental illness is that it is believed that such behavior is usually a defensive reaction to external stress: "[This condition] consists of varying degrees of conscious simulation of the previous psychotic state by and under the control of the patient's ego when a subsequent situation of stress occurs [Sadow and Sus-lick, 1961:452]." This psychiatric definition closely parallels Lemert's (1951) sociological definition "secondary deviation": "When a person begins to em-ploy his deviant behavior or a role based upon it as a means of defense, attack, or adjustment to the overt and covert problems created by the consequent societal reaction, his deviation is secondary [p. 76].'' Moreover, it appears that such simulation can occur even where there has been no previous psychotic episode:

> A particularly striking example of this was seen in a young hospital record custodian who developed a complex of subjective symptoms highly suggestive of a frontal lobe brain tumor. Laboratory and physical tests short of air studies had revealed that her difficulties were of a conversion-like nature and were in part patterned after case histories which she had read with more diligence than called for by her job [Sadow and Suslick, 1961:453].

Apparently, one can play the role of a mentally ill person without ever having actually experienced the role. Vicarious learning of imagery of the role of the mentally ill will be discussed shortly in the section following Proposition 5.

The Ganser syndrome appears to illustrate the intricate manner in which voluntary and involuntary elements intertwine in role-playing. This condition is referred to by psychiatrists as the ''approximate answer'' or *Vorbeireden* (talking past the point) syndrome:

> The patient is disoriented as to time and space and gives absurd answers to questions. Often he claims he does not know who he is, where he comes from, or where he is. When he is asked to do simple calculations, he makes obvious mistakes—for instance, giving 5 as the sum of 2 plus 2. When he is asked to identify objects, he gives the name of a related object. Upon being shown scissors, the patient may say they are knives; a picture of a dog may be identified as a cat, a yellow object may be called red, and so on. If he is asked what a hammer is used for, he may reply to cut wood. If he is shown a dime, he may state that it is a half dollar and so on. If he is asked how many legs a horse has, he may reply, ''Six.''
>
> At times almost a game seems to go on between the examiner and the patient. The examiner asks questions which are almost silly in their simplicity, but the patient succeeds in giving a sillier answer. And yet it seems that the patient undertands the question, because the answer, although wrong, is related to the question [Arieti and Meth, 1959:547].

In accordance with what has been said here about the social systemic nature of role-playing, the difficulty in interpreting simulation of previous psychotic states, and the Ganser syndrome, is that the patient is just as confused by his own behavior as is the observer.

Some psychiatrists suspect that in schizophrenia there is a large element of behavior that is in the borderline zone between volitional and nonvolitional activity. Here are some excerpts from an autobiographical account of schizophrenia which stress the role-playing aspects:

> We schizophrenics say and do a lot of stuff that is unimportant, and then we mix important things in with all this to see if the doctor cares enough to see them and feel them. . . .
>
> Patients laugh and posture when they see through the doctor who says he will help but really won't or can't. . . . They try to please the doctor but also confuse him so he won't go into anything important. When you find people who will really help, you don't need to distract them. You can act in a normal way.
>
> I can sense if the doctor not only wants to help but also can and will help. . . .
>
> Patients kick and scream and fight when they aren't sure the doctor can see them. It's a most terrifying feeling to realize that the doctor can't understand what you feel and that he's just

going ahead with his own ideas. I would start to feel that I was invisible or maybe not there at all. I had to make an uproar to see if the doctor would respond to me, not just his own ideas [Hayward and Taylor, 1956:211].

Note that this patient has applied to herself a deviant label ("we schizophrenics"), and that her behavior fits Lemert's definition of secondary deviation; she appears to have used the deviant role as a means of adjustment.

This discussion suggests that a stable role performance may arise when the actor's role imagery locks in with the type of "deference" that he regularly receives. An extreme example of this process may be taken from anthropological and medical reports concerning the "dead role," as in deaths attributed to "bone-pointing." Death from bone-pointing appears to arise from the conjunction of two fundamental processes that characterize all social behavior. First, all individuals continually orient themselves by means of responses that are perceived in social interaction: The individual's identity and continuity of experience are dependent on these cues.[3]

Generalizing from experimental findings, Blake and Mouton (1961) make this statement about the processes of conformity, resistance to influence, and conversion to a new role:

An individual requires a stable framework, including salient and firm reference points, in order to orient himself and to regulate his interactions with others. This framework consists of external and internal anchorages available to the individual whether he is aware of them or not. With an acceptable framework he can resist giving or accepting information that is inconsistent with the framework or that requires him to relinquish it. In the absence of a stable framework he actively seeks to establish one through his own strivings by making use of significant and relevant information provided within the context of interaction. By controlling the amount and kind of information available for orientation, he can be led to embrace conforming attitudes which are entirely foreign to his earlier ways of thinking [pp. 1–2].

Second, the individual has his own vocabulary of expectations, which may in a particular situation either agree with or be in conflict with the sanctions to which he is exposed. Entry into a role may be complete when this role is part of the individual's expectations and when these expectations are reaffirmed in social interaction. In the following pages, this principle is applied to the problem of the causation of mental disorder, through consideration of the social institution of insanity.

LEARNING AND MAINTAINING ROLE-IMAGERY

What are the beliefs and practices that constitute the social institution of insanity? And how do they figure in the development of mental disorder? Propositions 4 and 5 concerning beliefs about mental disorder in the general public are now considered.

[3]For a recent and striking demonstration of the effect of social communication in defining internal stimuli, see Schachter and Singer (1962).

Proposition 4: _Stereotyped imagery of mental disorder is learned in early childhood_. Although there are no substantiating studies in this area, scattered observations lead the author to conclude that children learn a considerable amount of imagery concerning deviance very early, and that much of the imagery comes from their peers rather than from adults. The literal meaning of _crazy_, a term now used in a wide variety of contexts, is probably grasped by children during the first years of elementary school. Since adults are often vague and evasive in their responses to questions in this area, an aura of mystery surrounds it. In this socialization, the grossest stereotypes that are heir to childhood fears (e.g., the "boogie man") survive. These conclusions are quite speculative, of course, and need to be investigated systematically, possibly with techniques similar to those used in studies of the early learning of racial stereotypes.

Here are a some psychiatric observations on "playing crazy" in a group of child patients (Cain, 1964). This material indicates that the social stereotypes are held by these children (ages 8–12) and play an active part in their cognition and behavior. It also fits the preceding discussion of role-playing and secondary deviation.

> Equally prominent are their intense concerns about craziness, about the possibility that _they themselves_ are crazy. . . . This concern seems to reflect the children's response to their own sporadic psychotic experience and behavior, a social awareness of how they appear to others, and perhaps in a sense an attempt to "explain" their own behavior. Undoubtedly, they are also reacting to teasing and name-calling by peers, and exasperated remarks by parents and teachers. . . .
>
> The child's concern about being crazy obtrudes in many different ways and places. Malcom, in associating to his figure drawing, perseverates remarks about craziness: "He's a crazy person," "He doesn't have a mind, just a nut," "A nut, that's the way he is, he was born that way," "She's nuts, that's what people say about her—Hitler was nuts, wasn't he?" Gale enters her therapist's office obviously upset, abruptly refuses to talk of any worries, insists she's fine. Soon she tells of seeing a sign in the waiting room about lectures on emotionally disturbed children, and she cries out that she's not crazy. Bob accidentally cuts his finger in the occupational therapy shop. Badly shaking, he stares at the blood and yells, "My God, I'm going crazy." Another talks of only wanting Looney Tunes comics: "Looney Tunes," he snorts, "that's for me all right." Mark finds he has confused his craft shop days, is afraid that this means he's losing his mind. Many of the children use humor about or project these concerns . . . describing . . . other people as "crazy." They often focus their craziness, with or without past neurological exams and EEG's, upon their brain—"Got no brain," "My brain is loose and swims around in my head," "My brain and mind are no good, they get tired too quick," "Sometimes I get—it feels like explosions in my head," "Something snaps up there."
>
> . . . A considerable component of the erratic behavior of these children has a conscious element—that is, they are "playing crazy." Much, though by no means all, of the playing crazy centers around their past experiences of and continual concerns about "being crazy." Their playing crazy takes many forms. It may be very quiet and subtle or blatant and obvious, identified as "pretend" by the child or exhaustively "defended" as crazy. Some of the varied forms are: "looking odd," staring off into space, or acting utterly confused; wild, primitive, disorganized ragelike states; odd verbalizations, incoherencies, mutterings; alleged hallucinations and delusions; the child's insistence that he is an animal, goblin, or other creature; or various grossly bizarre behaviors. Most of the children show many of these forms of playing

crazy. Most of the children make clear—though by no means reliable—announcements that they have played crazy or intend to do so, or speak of "just pretending." The complex components of their playing crazy often become clear only after extended observation and therapeutic work.

At times, the child is quite consciously, deliberately, almost zestfully playing crazy—he is under no significant internal pressure, is completely in control, and at the end is most reassured. For if one can openly *pretend* to be crazy, how can one really be crazy? Not only current concerns but actual past incidents may thus be magically wiped away. Perhaps more frequently, playing crazy is used as other types of play are often used, namely, to achieve belated mastery of traumatic events, or anxiety-provoking internal states. . . .

At still other times—again *not* when under much pressure or anywhere near disintegration— the children pretend or toy with craziness, in a deliberate and controlled manner, as if they were almost experimenting with or testing attenuated psychotic experiences: the behavior somehow seems directed toward mastery of anticipated states rather than toward reduction of old anxieties. One feels that the child is saying, "What if such-and-such should happen. . . ?." or "What would it be like if . . . ?" It might well be labeled an "antisurprise" measure, though clearly the previous psychotic states are not totally unrelated to this form of behavior, in which the child tentatively feels his way into feared future experiences of disintegration. Fenichel puts it well: ". . . a test action: repeating the overwhelming past and anticipating the possible future." Tensions are created, ". . . which *might* occur, but at a time and in a degree which is determined by the participant himself, and which is therefore under control."

At other times, when slipping toward or virtually in a psychotic state, the children may still attempt in a frenzied fashion to pretend to be crazy. Or perhaps more accurately, they pretend to be *crazier* than they are at that moment. . . .

Sometimes the child keeps a sharp eye on his audience's reaction while producing a quite contrived, controlled production of craziness. He fretfully awaits a response as he asks an observer to define him. "*Am* I insane? Do *you* think I'm so insane, so out of control that I could *really* . . . behave this way?" Should the response be oversolicitous, he may be badly threatened by the possibility that he *is* what he fears and pretends to be. And he may angrily plead, as did Bart on such occasions, "I'm not *that* crazy!" [pp. 280–282; footnotes omitted].

Assuming that Proposition 4 is sound, what effect does early learning have on the shared conceptions of insanity held in the community? In early childhood, much fallacious material is learned that is later discarded when more adequate information replaces it. This question leads to Proposition 5.

Proposition 5: *The stereotypes of insanity are continually reaffirmed, inadvertently, in ordinary social interaction.* Although many adults become acquainted with medical concepts of mental illness, the traditional stereotypes are not discarded but continue to exist alongside the medical conceptions, because the stereotypes receive almost continual support from the mass media and in ordinary social discourse. In mental health education campaigns, televised lectures by psychiatrists and others, magazine articles and newspaper feature stories, medical discussions of mental illness occur from time to time. These types of discussions, however, seem to be far outnumbered by stereotypic references.

A recent study by Nunnally (1961) demonstrates that the portrait of mental illness in mass media is highly stereotyped. In a systematic and large-scale content analysis of television, radio, newspapers, and magazines, he found an image of mental disorder presented that was overwhelmingly stereotyped.

Media presentations emphasized the bizarre symptoms of the mentally ill. For example, information relating to factor I (the conception that mentally ill persons look and act different from 'normal' people) was recorded 89 times. Of these, 88 affirm the factor, that is, indicated or suggested that people with mental health problems "look and act different;" only one item denied factor I. In television dramas, for example, the afflicted person often enters the scene staring glassy-eyed, with his mouth widely ajar, mumbling incoherent phrases or laughing uncontrollably. Even in what would be considered the milder disorders, neurotic phobias and obsessions, the afflicted person is presented as having bizarre facial expressions and actions [p. 74].

Of particular interest are the comparisons made between the imagery of mental disorder in the mass media, among mental health experts, and in the general public. In addition to the mass media analysis, data were collected from a group of psychiatrists and psychologists and from a sample drawn from the total population. The comparisons are summarized in Figure 4.1.

The solid line, representing the responses of the mental health experts, lies furthest to the left, in the direction of least stereotypy. The small circles—summarizing the findings in the study of the mass media—lie, for the most part,

how do you read this?!?!

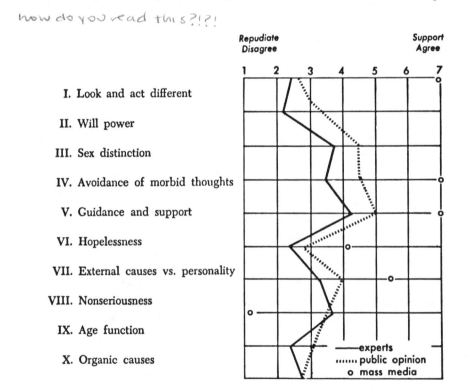

Fig. 4.1. Comparison of experts, the public, and the mass media on the 10 information factors (modified from Nunnally, 1961).

to the extreme right, the direction of greatest stereotypy. The broken line, indicating the findings of the sample survey in the public, lies between the mass media and the experts' profiles.

An interpretation of this finding is that the conceptions of mental disorder in the public are the resultant of cross-pressure: the opinions of experts, as expressed in mental health campaigns and "serious" mass media programming, pulling public opinion away from stereotypes, but with the more frequent and visible mass media productions reinforcing the traditional stereotypes.

Since Nunnally's sample of the mass media was taken during a single time period (1 week of 1955), he makes no direct analysis of trends in time. However, he does present some direct evidence which is quite relevant to this discussion. He presents the number of television programs dealing with mental illness and subdivides them into documentary programs, which are presumably serious medical discussions, as contrasted with other programs; that is, features and films for each year during the period 1951–1958. His findings are presented in Table 4.1

Once again, we see in a recent period (1957–1958) that the other features outnumber the serious programs with a ratio of the order of 100:1. Apparently, moreover, this disproportion was not decreasing, as many mental health workers believed, but actually increasing, as popular interest in mental disorder increases.

Although Nunnally's study represents a contribution to our knowledge of the imagery in the mass media and the general public, it is somewhat limited in terms of our present discussion, because the study deals only with direct references to mental illness and uses an incomplete set of categories for evaluating the references. The set of categories will be discussed first: Direct references are discussed shortly.

The categories that are used in evaluating the content of the imagery of mental illness are of unequal interest; Category 1 ("Look and act different") and category 6 ("hopelessness") are probably essential in understanding the mental illness imagery in the general public. There are other dimensions, however,

TABLE 1.   Number of Television Programs Dealing with Mental Illness, *1951–1958*[a]

	1951–53	*1954*	*1955*
Documentary programs	4	15	2
Other (features and films)	1	12	37
	1956	*1957*	*1958*
Documentary programs	2	1	1
Other (features and films)	122	169	72

[a]From Nunnally (1961).

which are not included in Nunnally's analysis, the most important of which are dangerousness, unpredictability, and negative evaluation. This can be made clear by referring to newspaper coverage of mental illness.

In newspapers it is a common practice to mention that a rapist or a murderer was once a mental patient. Here are several examples: Under the headline "Question Girl in Child Slaying," the story begins, "A 15-year-old girl *with a history of mental illness* is being questioned in connection with a kidnap–slaying of a 3-year-old boy." A similar story under the headline "Man Killed, Two Policemen Hurt in Hospital Fray," begins "*A former mental patient* grabbed a policeman's revolver and began shooting at 15 persons in the receiving room of City Hostpital No. 2 Thursday."

Often acts of violence will be connected with mental illness on the basis of little or no evidence. For instance, under the headline "Milwaukee Man Goes Berserk, Shoots Officer," the story describes the events and then quotes a police captain who said, "He may be a mental case." In another story, under the headline, "Texas Dad Kills Self, Four Children, Daughter Says," the last sentence of the story is "One report said Kinsey (the killer) was once a mental patient." In most large newspapers, there apparently is at least one such story in every issue.

Even if the coverage of these acts of violence was highly accurate, it would still give the reader a misleading impression, because negative information is seldom offset by positive reports. An item like the following is almost inconceivable: "Mrs. Ralph Jones, an ex-mental patient, was elected president of the Fairview Home and Garden Society at their meeting last Thursday."

Because of highly biased reporting, the reader is free to make the unwarranted inference that murder and rape and other acts of violence occur more frequently among former mental patients than among the population at large. Actually, it has been demonstrated that the incidence of crimes of violence (or of any crime) is much lower among former mental patients than in the general population.[4] Yet, because of newspaper practice, this is not the picture presented to the public. Newspapers have established an ineluctable relationship between mental illness and violence. Perhaps as importantly, this connection also signifies the incurability of mental disorder; that is, it connects *former* mental patients with violent and unpredictable acts.

It seems paradoxical that progress in communication techniques has created a situation in which the stereotyping process is probably growing stronger. News-

[4]H. Brill and B. Malzberg, Statistical Report Based on the Arrest Record of 5,354 ex-patients released from New York State Mental Hospitals during the period 1946–1948 (available from the authors). See also Cohen and Freeman (1945), Hastings (1958), and Rappeport *et al.* (1962). Suicide is an important exception to these findings. The rate of suicide is reported in a number of studies as considerably higher among patients and ex-patients than among the rest of the population. Even though the relative rate is high, the absolute rate is still quite low. For example, a recent study reports a suicide rate of 1.65% for patients and ex-patients of the psychiatric service of a Texas VA Hospital as compared with 0.23% for a comparable nonpatient group (Pokorny, 1964). W. O. Hagstrom suggested this exception to me.

papers now use teletype release from the press associations; and since these associations report incidents of crime and violence involving mental patients from the entire nation, the sampling bias in the picture presented to the public is enormous.

There are approximately 600,000 adults confined to mental hospitals in the United States on any 1 day, and an even larger group of former mental patients. The newspaper practice of daily reporting the violent acts of some patient, or former patient, and at the same time, seldom indicating the size of the vast group of nonviolent patients, is grossly misleading. Inadvertently, newspapers use selective reporting of the same type that is found in the most blatantly false advertisements and propaganda to continually "prove" that mental patients are unpredictably violent.

The impact of selective reportage is great because it confirms the public's stereotypes of insanity. Even if the newspaper were to explain the bias in these stories, the problem would not be eliminated. The vivid portrayal of a single case of human violence has more emotional impact on the reader than the statistics that indicate the true actuarial risks from mental patients as a class.

The average person's reaction to the fact that the probability of the kind of violence that the newspapers report occurring is about one in a million, is usually that this is still a real risk which he will not accept. Yet this is roughly the risk of death he unthinkingly accepts in taking a cross-country trip in an airplane or automobile. One component of the stereotype of insanity is an unreasoned and unreasonable fear of mental patients that makes the public reluctant to take risks in this area of the same size as risks frequently encountered and accepted in the ordinary round of living. *one is preventable, the other not, although it could be argued that the former shouldn't be preventable but obligatory*

Reaffirmation of the stereotype of insanity occurs not only in the mass media but indirectly in ordinary conversation: in jokes, anecdotes, and even in conventional phrases. Such phrases as "are you crazy?" or "it would be a madhouse," or "it's driving me out of my mind," or "we were chatting like crazy," or "he was running like mad," and literally hundreds of others occur frequently in informal conversations. In this usage, insanity itself is seldom the topic of conversation, and the discussants do not mean to refer to the topic of insanity and are usually unaware that they are doing so.

I have overheard mental patients, when talking among themselves, use these phrases unthinkingly. Even those mental health workers, such as psychiatrists, psychologists, and social workers, who are most interested in changing the concept of mental disorder often use these terms—sometimes jokingly but usually unthinkingly—in their informal discussions. These terms are so much a part of ordinary language that only the person who considers every word carefully can eliminate them from his speech. Through verbal usage, the stereotype of insanity is an inflexible part of the social structure.

The imagery which is implicit in these phrases should be discussed. When the phrase "running like mad" is used, the imagery which this conveys implicitly is movement of a wild and perhaps uncontrolled variety. The question "Are you out of your mind?" signifies a behavior of which the speaker disapproves. The

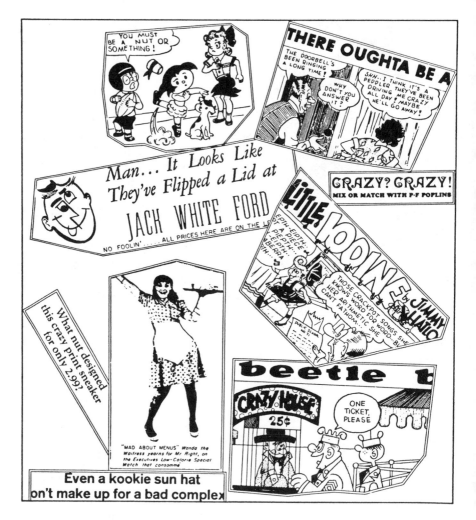

Fig. 4.2. Visual and verbal imagery about mental illness. (Clippings from newspapers and magazines.)

frequently used term *crazy*, often, although not always, implies subtle ridicule or stigma. These implications are there even when the person using the terms does not mean the words to convey this.

This inadvertent and incidental imagery is similar to that contained in racial and ethnic stereotypes. A speaker who uses the phrase, ''Jew a man down,'' may not necessarily be prejudiced against Jews (as in the rural South, where Jews are rare) but simply uses the phrase as a matter of convenience in order to convey his meaning; but to others, the assumptions are unmistakable—the image of the Jew as a person who is scheming and overinterested in money for its own sake.

Again as in racial and ethnic stereotypes, imagery is sometimes conveyed through jokes and anecdotes.[5] An example of the type of joke that one hears in informal conversation is taken from the *Reader's Digest*:

> A visitor to a mental hospital sees a patient who looks and acts like a normal person. He asks him why he is in the hospital. "Because I like potato pancakes," the patient replies. The visitor says, "That's nothing, I like potato pancakes myself." The patient turns to the visitor excitedly, "You do!" he replies, "Why don't you come to my room then, I have a whole trunkfull!"

The implications that one may draw from this type of joke are fairly clear. Persons who are mentally ill, even when they do not seem to be, are basically different. This is one theme, among others, which recurs in reference to mental illness in ordinary conversation. This theme, together with the "looks and acts different" theme and the "incurable" theme, is probably part of a single larger pattern: These deviants (like other deviants) belong to a fundamentally different class of human beings or perhaps even a different species. This is a manifestation of out-grouping, the beliefs and actions that are based on the premise that one's enemies, strangers, or deviants, no matter how attractive or sympathetic they may seem to the unwary, are essentially and fundamentally different from one's own kind.

A racial joke will provide an illustration of this genre, the fundamental difference and inferiority, of the outgroup:

> A Negro advertising executive is interviewed in his home, a luxurious apartment on the Hudson, on the television program Person-to-Person. He is impeccably dressed, articulate, and speaks with the easy, cultivated accents of East Coast society. He says, "Good evening Ed." Murrow says, "Good evening, Mr. Johnson." The executive introduces his family. Murrow says, "Before you take us on a tour of your home, could you tell our audience something about your working day? Mr. Johnson says, "Certainly, Ed. On the typical weekday, my man comes around to pick me up about 9, and we get to the Avenue about 10. I have an accounts conference until 12, lunch and cocktails till 2. At 2 another accounts conference until 4, then I dictate letters until about 6. My man picks me up, I'm home by 7. As often as not, we have people over for dinner and drinks. They stay until 11 or 12, then I go out on the balcony, and *jes look out ober de ribber*."

To summarize this section: public stereotypes of mental illness are difficult to change because they receive continual although inadvertent support from the mass media and in ordinary conversation. In support of this proposition, evidence from several studies and the author's observations have been cited.

On the basis of this evidence, one would suspect that mental health campaigns which are based largely on disseminating information will be doomed to failure because of the overwhelming preponderance of stereotyped information and imagery to which the average person is exposed.

---

[5]For references to the use of humor as an instrument of social control, see Middleton and Moland (1959).

It is difficult to say at this time how the situation could be changed. In some media, television for example, a definite attempt is made to "clean up" the references to mental illness. As Nunnally (1961) points out, however, these attempts are not particularly successful. While television has managed to eliminate virtually all the irreverent slang references to mental illness such as "goof ball," "flipped," "nut," and "loony," there has been no attempt to change the visual imagery.

Why are these stereotypes resistant to change? One possible explanation is that they are functional for the current social order and tend to be integrated into the psychological make-up of all members of the society. Racial stereotypes may perform similar functions. In the southern part of the United States, for example, racial stereotypes are not fortuitous and isolated attitudes; rather, they are integral parts of the southerner's cognitive structure. The stereotype of the Negro fulfills the functions of a contrast conception, a reference point for making social comparisons and self-evaluations. One clue to the existence of contrast conceptions is a highly proliferated vocabulary of vernacular terms, such as exists in the South for referral to Negroes. "Jig," "coon," "spade," "buck," and "jungle bunny" are only a few of an enormous number of such terms. In current vernacular, there is an equally large number of terms for referring to insanity, or going insane; a few specimens are: "out of one's mind," or "losing one's mind," or "the mind snapping," "out of one's head," "wrong in the head," "not right in the head," (or a gesture in which one moves the finger in a circle while pointing to one's head), "teched in the head," "cracked," "loony," "off one's rocker," "off the deep end," "nuts," "bughouse," "flipped," "psycho," "goofy," "ga-ga," "lose your marbles," "bats in the belfry" (or just "bats"), "screwy" or "screwball," "crazy," "deranged," "demented," and others.

Judging from the frequency with which references to mental disorder appear in the mass media and in colloquial speech, the concept of *mental disorder* serves as a fundamental contrast conception in our society, functioning to preserve the current mores. The displacement of such a convenient concept is probably resisted for this reason. In some preliterate societies, the concept of *spirit possession* "explains" dreams, sickness, mental disorder, great success, untimely death, and many otherwise unexplainable phenomena. The average member of such a society has, therefore, a substantial psychological investment in the belief in spirit possession.

Similarly, in the United States, the average citizen resists changes in his concept of insanity—or, if he is in the middle class, his concept of mental disease—because these concepts are functional for maintaining his customary moral and congitive world.

This section concludes with a discussion of a process which may relate stereotyping of the mentally ill to the social dynamics of mental illness: vicarious learning. The transmission of stereotyped imagery in the mass media and ordinary conversation may throw light on a question that has been hotly debated;

whether the symptoms of mental disorder are inherent or learned. Although advocates of the learning point of view have pointed to instances where symptoms seemed to be learned (*foie à deux*, role models in the family), they have never been completely satisfied with this explanation, since it places so much emphasis on what seems to be infrequent occurrences.

The discussion here suggests that *everyone* in a society learns the symptoms of mental disorder vicariously through the imagery that is conveyed, unintentionally, in everyday life. This imagery tends to be tied to the vernacular of each language and culture; this association may be one reason why there are considerable variations in the symptoms of mental disorder that occur in different cultures. If, as suggested here, this imagery is available to the rule-breaker to structure and thus to "understand" his own experience, the quality of the societal reaction becomes extremely important in determining the duration and outcome of the initially amorphous and unstructured residual rule-breaking. The nature of the societal reaction is shown in the next section to be made up of alternative, indeed, mutually exclusive components—normalization or labeling.

NORMALIZATION AND LABELING

According to the analysis presented here, the traditional stereotypes of mental disorder are solidly entrenched in the population because they are learned early in childhood and are continuously reaffirmed in the mass media and in everyday conversation. How do these beliefs function in the processes leading to mental disorder? This question is considered first by referring to the earlier discussion of the societal reaction to residual rule-breaking.

It was stated that the usual reaction to residual rule-breaking is normalization and that in these cases most rule-breaking is transitory. The societal reaction to rule-breaking is not always normalization, however. In a small proportion of cases, the reaction goes the other way, exaggerating and at times distorting the extent and degree of the violation. This pattern or exaggeration, which we will call "labeling," has been noted by Garfinkel (1956) in his discussion of the "degradation" of officially recognized criminals. Goffman (1961) makes a similar point in his description of the "discrediting" of mental patients.

> (The patient's case record) is apparently not regularly used to record occasions when the patient showed capacity to cope honorably and effectively with difficult life situations. Nor is the case record typically used to provide a rough average of sampling of his past conduct. (Rather, it extracts) from his whole life course a list of those incidents that have or might have had "symptomatic" significance. . . . I think that most of the information gathered in case records is quite true, although it might seem also to be true that almost anyone's life course could yield up enough denigrating facts to provide grounds for the record's justification of commitment.

Apparently under some conditions, the societal reaction to rule-breaking is to seek out signs of abnormality in the deviant's history to show that he was always essentially a deviant.

The contrasting social reactions of normalization and labeling provides a means of answering two fundamental questions. First, if rule-breaking arises from diverse sources—physical, psychological, and situational—how does the uniformity of behavior that is associated with insanity develop? Second, if rule-breaking is usually transitory, how does it become stabilized in those patients who become chronically deviant? To summarize, what are the sources of uniformity and stability of deviant behavior?

In the approach taken here, the answer to this question is based on Propositions 4 and 5, that the role imagery of insanity is learned early in childhood and is reaffirmed in social interaction. In a crisis, when the deviance of an individual becomes a public issue, the traditional stereotype of insanity becomes the guiding imagery for action, both for those reacting to the deviant and, at times, for the deviant himself. When societal agents and persons around the deviant react to him uniformly in terms of the traditional stereotypes of insanity, his amorphous and unstructured rule-breaking tends to crystallize in conformity to these expectations, thus becoming similar to the behavior of other deviants classified as mentally ill, and stable over time. The process of becoming uniform and stable is completed when the traditional imagery becomes a part of the deviant's orientation for guiding his own behavior.

The idea that cultural stereotypes may stabilize residual rule-breaking and tend to produce uniformity in symptoms, is supported by cross-cultural studies of mental disorder. Although some observers insist there are underlying similarities, many agree that there are enormous differences in the manifest symptoms of stable mental disorder *between* societies and great similarity *within* societies (Yap, 1951).

These considerations suggest that the labeling process is a crucial contingency in most careers of residual deviance. Thus Glass (1953), who observed that neuropsychiatric casualities may not become mentally ill if they are kept with their unit, goes on to say that military experience with psychotherapy has been disappointing. Soldiers who are removed from their unit to a hospital, he states, often go on to become chronically impaired.[6] That is, their deviance is stabilized by the labeling process, which is implicit in their removal and hospitalization. A similar interpretation can be made by comparing the observations of childhood disorders among Mexican–Americans with those of "Anglo" children. Childhood disorders such as *susto* (an illness believed to result from fright) sometimes have damaging outcomes in Mexican–American children (Saunders, 1954:142). Yet the deviant behavior involved is very similar to that which seems to have high incidence among Anglo children, with permanent impairment virtually never occurring. Apparently through cues from his elders, the Mexican–American child, behaving initially much like his Anglo counterpart, learns to enter the sick role, at times with serious consequences.[7]

---

[6]For a contrary view, see Ginzberg (1959).

[7]For a discussion, with many illustrative cases, of the process in which persons play the "dead role" and subsequently die, see Herbert (1961).

ACCEPTANCE OF THE DEVIANT ROLE

From this point of view, most mental disorder can be considered to be a social role. This social role complements and reflects the status of the insane in the social structure. It is through the social processes which maintain the status of the insane that the varied rule-breaking from which mental disorder arises is made uniform and stable. The stabilization and uniformization of residual deviance are completed when the deviant accepts the role of the insane as the framework within which he organizes his own behavior. Three propositions are stated below which suggest some of the processes which cause the deviant to accept such a stigmatized role.

Proposition 6: *Labeled deviants may be rewarded for playing the stereotyped deviant role.* Ordinarily patients who display "insight" are rewarded by psychiatrists and other personnel. That is, patients who manage to find evidence of "their illness" in their past and present behavior, confirming the medical and societal diagnosis, receive benefits. This pattern of behavior is a special case of a more general pattern that has been called the "apostolic function" by Balint (1957), in which the physician and others inadvertently cause the patient to display symptoms of the illness the physician thinks the patient has. The apostolic function occurs in the context of bargaining between the patient and the doctor over what shall be decided to be the nature of the patient's illness:

> Some of the people who, for some reason or other, find it difficult to cope with problems of their lives resort to becoming ill. If the doctor has the opportunity of seeing them in the first phases of their being ill, i.e. before they settle down to a definite "organized" illness, he may observe that these patients, so to speak, offer or propose various illnesses, and that they have to go on offering new illnesses until between doctor and patient an agreement can be reached resulting in the acceptance by both of them of one of the illnesses as justified [p. 18].

It is in this fluid situation that Balint believes the doctor influences the manifestations of illness:

> Apostolic mission or function means in the first place that every doctor has a vague, but almost unshakably firm, idea of how a patient ought to behave when ill. Although this idea is anything but explicit and concrete, it is immensely powerful, and influences, as we have found, practically every detail of the doctor's work with his patients. *It was almost as if every doctor had revealed knowledge of what was right and what was wrong for patients to expect and to endure, and further, as if he had a sacred duty to convert to his faith all the ignorant and unbelieving among his patients* [p. 216].

Not only physicians but other hospital personnel and even other patients, reward the deviant for conforming to the stereotypes. Caudill (1952), who made observations of ward life in the guise of being a patient, reports various pressures from fellow patients. In the following excerpt, for example, there is the suggestion in the advice of the other patients that he should realize that he is a sick man:

On the second day, following a conference with his therapist, the observer expressed resentment over not having going-out privileges to visit the library and work on his book—his compulsive concern over his inability to finish this task being (according to his simulated case history) one of the factors leading to his hospitalization. Immediately two patients, Mr. Hill and Mrs. Lewis, who were later to become his closest friends, told him he was being "defensive"; since his doctor did not wish him to do such work, it was probably better "to lay off it." Mr. Hill went on to say that one of his troubles when he first came to the hospital was thinking of things that he had to do or thought he had to do. He said that now he did not bother about anything. Mrs. Lewis said that at first she had treated the hospital as a sort of hotel and had spent her therapeutic hours "charming" her doctor, but it had been pointed out to her by others that this was a mental hospital and that she should actively work with her doctor if she expected to get well [p. 314–344].

In the California mental hospital in which the author conducted a study in 1959, a common theme in the discussions between patients on the admissions wards was the "recognition" of one's illness. This interchange, which took place during a ward meeting on a female admission ward, provides an extreme example:

NEW PATIENT: "I don't belong here. I don't like all these crazy people. When can I talk to the doctor? I've been here four days and I haven't seen the doctor. I'm not crazy."

ANOTHER PATIENT: "She says she's not crazy." (Laughter from patients.)

ANOTHER PATIENT: "Honey, what I'd like to know is, if you're not crazy, how did you get your ass in this hospital?"

NEW PATIENT: "It's complicated, but I can explain. My husband and I. . . ."

FIRST PATIENT: "That's what they all say." (General Laughter.)

Thus there is considerable pressure on the patient to accept the role of the mentally ill as part of this self-conception.

Proposition 7: *Labeled deviants are punished when they attempt the return to conventional roles.* The second process operative is the systematic blockage of entry to nondeviant roles once the label has been publicly applied.[8] Thus the former mental patient, although he is urged to rehabilitate himself in the community, usually finds himself discriminated against in seeking to return to his old status and on trying to find a new one in the occupational, marital, social, and other spheres.

Recent studies have shown that former mental patients, like ex-convicts may find it difficult to find employment, even when their behavior and qualifications are unexceptional. In an experimental study, Phillips (1963) has shown that the rejection of the mentally ill is largely a matter of stigmatization, rather than an evaluation of their behavior.

Despite the fact that the "normal" person is more an "ideal type" than a normal person, when he is described as having been in a mental hospital he is rejected more than psychotic individuals described as not seeking help or as seeing a clergyman, and more than a depressed-

---

[8]Lemert (1951) provides an extensive discussion of this process under the heading, "Limitation of Participation," pp. 434–440.

neurotic seeing a clergyman. Even when the normal person is described as (only) seeing a psychiatrist, he is rejected more than a simple schizophrenic who seeks no help, (and) more than a phobic-compulsive individual seeking no help or seeing a clergyman or physician [p. 963–973].

Propositions 6 and 7, taken together, suggest that to a degree the labeled deviant is rewarded for deviating and punished for attempting to conform.

Proposition 8: *In the crisis occurring when a residual rule-breaker is publicly labeled, the deviant is highly suggestible and may accept the proffered role of the insane as the only alternative.* When gross rule-breaking is publicly recognized and made an issue, the rule-breaker may be profoundly confused, anxious, and ashamed. In this crisis, it seems reasonable to assume that the rule-breaker will be suggestible to the cues that he gets from the reactions of others toward him.[9] But those around him are also in a crisis; the incomprehensible nature of the rule-breaking, and the seeming need for immediate action lead them to take collective action against the rule-breaker on the basis of the attitude which all share—the traditional stereotypes of insanity. The rule-breaker is sensitive to the cues provided by these others and begins to think of himself in terms of the stereotyped role of insanity, which is part of his own role vocabulary also, since he, like those reacting to him, learned it early in childhood. In this situation, his behavior may begin to follow the pattern suggested by his own stereotypes and the reactions of others. That is, when a residual rule-breaker organizes his behavior within the framework of mental disorder, and when his organization is validated by others, particularly prestigeful others such as physicians, he is "hooked" and will proceed on a career of chronic deviance.

There is little direct evidence for the part played by role-images in the development of mental illness, but there are various suggestions that it may be an important one. For example, Rogler and Hollingshead (1965), in their study of schizophrenia in Puerto Rico, give considerable emphasis to the role of the *loco* (lunatic) in the cases they studied. Comparing the 40 persons diagnosed as schizophrenic with the control group, they state:

> The role of the *loco* presents a problem to nearly all schizophrenic persons but to only a few who are free of the illness. Sick persons are extraordinarily defensive about the topic of the loco. Time and again, they state that they are not *locos* when no such question is being asked. When asked directly, only one sick person states that he is a *loco*; only one spouse of a sick person asserts this of his mate. The remaining persons in the sick group do not admit to *locura*. Rather, after a forceful denial, they add such phrases as: "Sometimes I act like one, but I am not one." "I may eventually become one, but I am not one now." "If I don't get help, I may become *loco*." "Perhaps I am on the road to becoming one." "Only at times do I act like a *loco* [p. 221].

Although all but 2 of the 40 persons diagnosed as schizophrenic denied being *loco* in response to direct questions, the fact that they themselves raised the issue

[9]This proposition receives support from Erikson's observations (1957).

when the question was not asked suggests that the role image of the *loco* was being used in their own thought processes, regardless of their explicit denial. It is important for the reader to understand that the diagnosis of schizophrenia was made as part of the research process in this study and not necessarily officially in the community. The subjects were persons who had sought psychiatric help, and who were diagnosised as schizophrenic by a psychiatrist attached to the research group. From the point of view presented here, we may consider the "sick" (i.e., schizophrenic) group as persons who are experimenting with the role of the mentally ill.

Rogler and Hollingshead (1965) also found that the role image of the *loco* held by the "sick" group was not different from that held by the rest of the community.

> Schizophrenic persons are particularly vulnerable to being assigned the role of the *loco*. Consequently, we explored the possibility that the schizophrenic's portrayal of this role would be drawn in less harsh and more benign terms than that drawn by well people. This idea was erroneous! There is no tendency on the part of the schizophrenics to soften the portrait of the *loco*; sick and well persons describe him as violent, immoral, criminal, filthy, idiosyncratic, and worthless. Moreover, men and women do not differ in their conceptions of the *loco*. Their views are uniform and deep; perhaps they are fixed unalterably [p. 218].

This finding is in accord with Propositions 4 and 5: if deviant role imagery is learned early and continually reaffirmed, a person's image of insanity would not be likely to be affected even when he himself runs the risk of being labeled. The role images are integral parts of the social structure and therefore not easily relinquished. Holding these relatively fixed images, the rule-breaker, like those around him, is susceptible to social suggestion in a crisis.

The role of suggestion is noted by Warner (1958) in his description of bone-pointing magic:

> The effect of (the suggestion of the entire community on the victim) is obviously drastic. An analogous situation in our society is hard to imagine. If all a man's near kin, his father, mother, brothers and sisters, wife, children, business associates, friends, and all the other members of the society, should suddenly withdraw themselves because of some dramatic circumstance, refusing to take any attitude but one of taboo . . . and then perform over him a sacred ceremony . . . the enormous suggestive power of this movement . . . of the community after it has had its attitudes (toward the victim) crystallized can be somewhat understood by ourselves [p. 242].

If we substitute for black magic the taboo that usually accompanies mental disorder and consider a commitment proceeding or even mental hospital admission as a sacred ceremony, the similarity between Warner's description and the typical events in the development of mental disorder is considerable.

The last three propositions suggest that once a person has been placed in a deviant status, there are rewards for conforming to the deviant role and punishment for not conforming to the deviant role. This is not to imply, however, that the symptomatic behavior of persons occupying a deviant status is always a manifestation of conforming behavior. To explain this point, some discussion of the process of self-control in "normals" is necessary.

In a recent discussion of the process of self-control, Shibutani (1961, Chapter 6) notes that self-control is not automatic but is an intricate and delicately balanced process, sustainable only under propitious circumstances. He points out that fatigue, the reaction to narcotics, excessive excitement or tension (such as is generated in mobs), or a number of other conditions interfere with self-control; conversely, conditions which produce normal bodily states, and deliberative processes, such as symbolization and imaginative rehearsal before action, facilitate it.

One may argue that a crucially important aspect of imaginative rehearsal is the image of himself that the actor projects into his future action. Certainly in American society, the cultural image of the "normal" adult is that of a person endowed with self-control ("will power," "backbone," or "strength of character"). For the person who sees himself as endowed with the trait of self-control, self-control is facilitated, since he can imagine himself enduring stress during his imaginative rehearsal and also while under actual stress.

For a person who has acquired an image of himself as lacking the ability to control his own actions, the process of self-control is likely to break down under stress. Such a person may feel that he has reached his "breaking-point" under circumstances which would be endured by a person with a "normal" self-conception. This is to say, a greater lack of self-control than can be explained by stress tends to appear in those roles for which the culture transmits imagery which emphasizes lack of self-control. In American society, such imagery is transmitted for the roles of the very young and very old, drunkards and drug addicts, gamblers, and the mentally ill.

Thus, the social role of the mentally ill has a different significance at different phases of residual deviance. When labeling first occurs, it merely gives a name to rule-breaking which has other roots. When (and if) the rule-breaking becomes an issue and is not ignored or rationalized away, labeling may create a social type, a pattern of "symptomatic" behavior in conformity with the stereotyped expectations of others. Finally, to the extent that the deviant role becomes a part of the deviant's self-conception, his ability to control his own behavior may be impaired under stress, resulting in episodes of compulsive behavior.

The preceding eight hypotheses form the basis for the final causal hypothesis.

Proposition 9: _Among residual rule-breakers, labeling is among the most important causes of careers of residual deviance._ This proposition assumes that most residual rule-breaking, if it does not become the basis for entry into the sick role, will not lead to a deviant career.[10] The most usual case, according to the

---

[10]Sociologically, an occupational career can be defined as "the sequence of movements from one position to another in an occupational system made by any individual who works in that system" (Becker, 1963:24). Similarly, a deviant career is the sequence of movements from one stigmatized position to another in the sector of the larger social system that functions to maintain social control. For example, the frequently cited progression of young men from probation through detention centers and reform schools to prison, with intervening times spent out of prison, may be considered as recurring deviant career. For Becker's discussion of deviant careers, _see_ pp. 25–39.

argument that has been advanced here, is that there will be few if any social consequences of residual rule-breaking. Occasionally, however, such rule-breaking may become the basis for major changes in the rule-breaker's social status, other than demotion to the status of a mental patient. The three excerpts that follow illustrate such shifts.

CASE 1: Some of the Indian tribes of California accorded prestige principally to those who passed through certain trance experiences. Not all of these tribes believed that it was exclusively women who were so blessed, but among the Shasta this was the convention. Their shamans were women, and they were accorded the greatest prestige in the community. They were chosen because of their constitutional liability to trance and allied manifestations. One day the woman who was so destined, while she was about her usual work, fell suddenly to the ground. She had heard a voice speaking to her in tones of the greatest intensity. Turning, she had seen a man with drawn bow and arrow. He commanded her to sing on pain of being shot through the heart by his arrow, but under the stress of the experience she fell senseless. Her family gathered. She was lying rigidly, hardly breathing. They knew that for some time she had had dreams of a special character which indicated a shamanistic calling, dreams of escaping grizzly bears, falling off cliffs or trees, or of being surrounded by swarms of yellow-jackets. The community knew therefore what to expect. After a few hours the woman began to moan gently and to roll about upon the ground, trembling violently. She was supposed to be repeating the song which she had been told to sing and which during the trance had been taught her by the spirit itself, and immediately blood oozed from her mouth.

When the woman had come to herself after the first encounter with her spirit, she danced that night her first initiatory shaman's dance. For three nights she danced, holding herself by a rope that was swung from the ceiling. On the third night she had to receive in her body her power from the spirit. She was dancing, and as she felt the approach of the moment she called out, "He will shoot me, he will shoot me," Her friends stood close, for when she reeled in a kind of cataleptic seizure, they had to seize her before she fell or she would die. . . . From this time on she continued to validate her supernatural power by further cataleptic demonstrations, and she was called upon in great emergencies of life and death, for curing and for divination and for counsel. She became in other words, by this procedure a woman of great power and importance [Benedict, 1946:245–247].

CASE 2: [Samuel lived in the house of Eli, the priest. One night, as Samuel lay down, he heard a voice call his name] . . . and he answered, "Here am I." And he ran to Eli, and said, "Here am I; for thou callest me." And he said, "I called not; lie down again." And he went and lay down.

[Again Samuel heard his name called] . . . and Samuel arose and went to Eli, and said, "Here am I; for thou didst call me." And he answered, "I called not, my son; lie down again." [For the third time, Samuel heard his name called] . . . And he arose and went to Eli, and said, "Here am I, for thou didst call me." And Eli perceived that the Lord had called the child.

Therefore Eli said unto Samuel, "Go, lie down: and it shall be, if He call thee, that you shall say, Speak, Lord; for Thy servant heareth." So Samuel went and lay down in his place.

And the Lord came, and stood, and called as at other times, "Samuel, Samuel." Then Samuel answered, "Speak, Lord, for Thy servant heareth." [Samuel hears prophesized the downfall of the house of Eli] . . . And all Israel from Dan even to Beersheba knew that Samuel was established to be a prophet of the Lord. [1 Sam. 3:4–6, 8–10, 20].

CASE 3: INTERVIEWER: "How did you first come to believe that you had psychic powers?"
MRS. BENDIT: ". . . during this particular period of my life, I was facing a number of personal

problems that seemed overwhelming to me at the time. I was thoroughly depressed and confused, and I felt that the strain was getting progressively worse. I had been in this state for abut two weeks, when one Sunday morning, in church, I was shocked to see, up in the rafters of the ceiling of the church, a group of angels. I couldn't keep my eyes from the sight, although I noticed that no one else in the congregation was looking up. After this experience, I wandered around for several days, hardly knowing what to do with myself. One evening soon after, I went to a reception, hoping to take my mind from my troubles.

"I stayed pretty much to myself at the party, but I soon noticed, that across the room there was a woman who was watching me intently. She finally came over to me and introduced herself. She then explained clairvoyance to me at some length. I told her about my vision in the church, She explained that this experience was an example of my psychic powers. She said that she was a psychic, and that she could tell that I had the gift also. Although her explanation sounded strange to me, I felt somewhat relieved. In the ensuing weeks, I saw her often and we had lengthy conversations. She introduced me into the group of clairvoyants and interested persons that she belonged to. . . . It was to this group that I first began to demonstrate my clairvoyance. . . . Several years after this I was able to arrange, with the help of my husband [her husband is a physician] an appearance before the Royal Academy of Medicine for a demonstration of clairvoyance."[11]

Cases 1 and 2 illustrate elevations in social status that are based on primary rule-breaking. Case 3 illustrates what may be called a lateral movement in status, since Mrs. Bendit has obviously become completely identified with her role as a clairvoyant.

The likelihood that residual rule-breaking in itself will not lead to labeling as a deviant draws attention to the central significance of the contingencies that influence the direction and intensity of the societal reaction. One of the urgent conceptual tasks for a sociological theory of deviant behavior is the development of a precise and widely applicable set of such contingencies. The classification that is offered here is only a crude first step in this direction.

Although there are a wide variety of contingencies which lead to labeling, they can be simply classified in terms of the nature of the rule-breaking, the person who breaks the rules, and the community in which the rule-breaking occurs. Other things being equal, the severity of the societal reaction is a function of first, the degree, amount, and visibility of the rule-breaking; second, the power of the rule-breaker and the social distance between him and the agents of social control; and finally, the tolerance level of the community and the availability in the culture of the community of alternative nondeviant roles.[12] Particularly crucial for future research is the importance of the first two contingencies (the amount and degree of rule-breaking), which are characteristics of the rule-breaker, relative to the remaining five contingencies, which are characteristics of the social system.[13] To the extent that these five factors are found empirically to be independent determinants of labeling and denial, the status of the mental

---

[11]Interview on radio station KPFA, Berkeley, California as recollected by the author.

[12]Cf. Lemert (1951:51–53, 55–68); Goffman (1961:134–135); Mechanic (1962). For a list of similar factors in the reaction to physical illness, see Koos (1954:30–38).

[13]Cf. Dinitz, Lefton, Angrist, and Pasamanick (1961) and Study II in Chapter 5.

patient can be considered a partly ascribed rather than a completely achieved status. The dynamics of treated mental illness could then be profitably studied quite apart from the individual dynamics of mental disorder by focusing on social systemic contingencies.

A NOTE ON FEEDBACK IN DEVIANCE-AMPLIFYING SYSTEMS

It should be noted, however, that these contingencies are causal only because they become part of a dynamic system: the reciprocal and cumulative interrelation between the rule-breaker's behavior and the social reaction.[14] For example, the more the rule-breaker enters the role of the mentally ill, the more he is defined by others as mentally ill; but the more he is defined as mentally ill, the more fully he enters the role, and so on. This kind of vicious circle is quite characteristic of may different kinds of social and individual systems. It is very important to understand the part that social contingencies play in such a system, since the cause–effect relationship is not a simple one.

In the Rogler and Hollingshead (1965) study of schizophrenia in Puerto Rico, the authors drew attention to the dynamic interrelation between role entry and changes in the deviant's self-conception.

> Although the sick person is deeply absorbed in his illness and yearns to speak about it, confidants are carefully selected. The illness is suppressed as a topic of conversation with friends and associates. Efforts are made to pretend that he is not a *loco*. He controls activities which exacerbate his *loco*-like behavior. These efforts are relatively futile, however, as the symptoms of the illness are strong and readily visible in the crowded social setting in which he lives. In point of fact, the sick person has begun to be viewed and treated as a *loco*. He withdraws from society out of fear that he will be stigmatized as a *loco*. In turn, the rejection by his friends and associates pushes him to withdraw. The stigma attached to this role is so strong that the withdrawal of the sick person from participation in all types of social groups appears to be a natural sequel to the condemnation he suffers [pp. 241–242].

The process described in this passage can be interpreted as a vicious circle begun by stigmatization, withdrawal to avoid more stigma, stigmatization because of withdrawal or its effects, and so on around the circle.

The vicious circle effect occurs not only in the entrance to role-playing by the rule-breaker but in other parts of the system also. In order to see this more clearly, it is useful to represent the theory as a flow chart (Figure 4.3).[15]

This chart makes it clear that the theory of stable mental disorder discussed here is actually an assembly of system modules which intereact. There is the module of residual rule-breaking, the contingency module which filters out most of the rule-breakers through denial, the crisis module, the rule-breaker's self-conception module, the social control module, which operates such that the

---

[14]For an explicit treatment of feedback, see Lemert (1962)

[15]W. Buckley suggested the use of this flow chart and provided help in interpreting the theory in cybernetic terms. For comment by Buckley, see his "Methodological Note" in the Appendix.

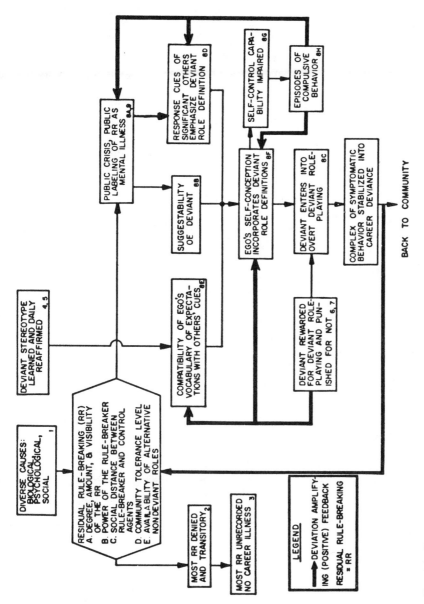

Fig. 4.3. Flow chart—indicating stabilization of deviance in a social system. (Heavy line indicates deviation amplifying [positive] feedback; residual rule-breaking-RR.)

deviant tends to play the stereotyped deviant role, and finally, the compulsive behavior module. Each of these modules is a system in itself with its own contingencies. In the context of the larger theory, however, each is a subsystem, which under proper conditions, operates as part of the entire network.

The total system forms what Maruyama has called a "deviation-amplifying system," in which low probability events are stabilized. In such a system, the simple causal laws in which similar conditions of deviance produce similar effects is not operative. Even more complicated models of contingent cause do not work, because it is necessary to specify the state of the entire system.

In cybernetic terms, what we have referred to as a vicious circle is called positive feedback, and it is apparent from the chart that there are a number of feedback loops in the system. The episodes of compulsive behavior interact with the earlier crisis, other's responses, and the deviant's self-conception sub-systems, and the playing of the deviant role feeds back to the system of social control and the deviant's self-conception as well. Under proper conditions, deviation is not damped out by the action of the system, which is the usual situation in social systems, but is stabilized or even amplified.

CONCLUSION

The discussion to this point has presented a sociological theory of the causation of stable mental disorder. Since the evidence advanced in support of the theory was scattered and fragmentary, it can only be suggested as a stimulus to further discussion and research. Among the areas pointed out for further investigation are field studies of the prevalence and duration of residual rule-breaking; investigations of stereotypes of mental disorder in children, the mass media, and adult conversations; studies of the rewarding of stereotyped deviation, blockage of return to conventional roles, and of the suggestibility of rule-breakers in crises. The final causal hypothesis suggests studies of the conditions under which normalization and labeling of residual rule-breaking occur. The variable that may effect the societal reaction concern the nature of the rule-breaking, the rule-breaker himself, and the community in which the rule-breaking occurs. Although many of the propositions suggested are largely unverified, they suggest avenues for investigating mental disorder different from those that are usually followed and the rudiments of a general theory of deviant behavior. In Chapter 5 a study of hospitalization and release based upon this theory is described.

II
Research

Decisions in Medicine[1]

5

THE discussion to this point has concerned a theory of stable mental illness. In this chapter and the following chapter, our attention shifts from theory to practice. In Chapter 6, two studies of psychiatric decision making are reported which are relevant to our theoretical concerns. This chapter introduces the studies in Chapter 6 by a discussion of a decision-making problem that psychiatry shares with general medicine. Members of professions such as law and medicine frequently are confronted with uncertainty in the course of their routine duties. In these circumstances, informal norms have developed for handling uncertainty so that paralyzing hesitation is avoided. These norms are based upon assumptions that some types of error are more to be avoided than others—assumptions so basic that they are usually taken for granted, are seldom discussed, and are therefore slow to change.

The purpose of this chapter is to describe one important norm for handling uncertainty in medical diagnosis, that judging a sick person well is more to be avoided than judging a well person sick, and to suggest some of the consequences of the application of this norm in medical practice. Apparently this norm, like many important cultural norms, "goes without saying" in the subculture of the medical profession; in form, however, it resembles any decision

[1]An earlier version of this chapter was presented as a paper at the Conference on Mathematical Models in the Behavioral and Social Sciences, sponsored by the Western Management Science Institute, University of California at Los Angeles, Cambria, California, 1961.

rule for guiding behavior under conditions of uncertainty. In the discussion that follows, decision rules in law, statistics, and medicine are compared in order to indicate the types of error that are thought to be the more important to avoid and the assumptions underlying this preference. On the basis of recent findings of the widespread distribution of elements of disease and deviance in normal populations, the assumption of a uniform relationship between disease signs and impairment is criticized. Finally, it is suggested that to the extent that physicians are guided by this medical decision rule, they too often place patients in the ''sick role'' who could otherwise have continued in their normal pursuits.

To the extent that physicians and the public are biased toward treatment, the ''creation'' of illness (i.e., the production of unnecessary impairment) may go hand in hand with the prevention and treatment of disease in modern medicine. The magnitude of the bias toward treatment in any single case may be quite small, since there are probably other medical decision rules (''When in doubt, delay your decision'') which counteract the rule discussed here. Even a small bias, however, if it is relatively constant throughout Western society, can have effects of large magnitude. Since this argument is based largely on fragmentary evidence, it is intended merely to stimulate further discussion and research rather than to demonstrate the validity of a point of view. The discussion begins with the consideration of a decision rule in law.

In criminal trials in England and the United States, there is an explicit rule for arriving at decisions in the face of uncertainty: ''A man is innocent until proven guilty.'' The meaning of this rule is made clear by the English common-law definition of the phrase ''proven guilty,'' which, according to tradition, is that the judge or jury must find the evidence of guilt compelling *beyond a reasonable doubt*. The basic legal rule for arriving at a decision in the face of uncertainty may be briefly stated: ''When in doubt, acquit.'' That is, the jury or judge must not be equally wary of erroneously convicting or acquitting: the error that is most important to avoid is to erroneously convict. This concept is expressed in the maxim, ''Better a thousand guilty men go free, than one innocent man be convicted.''

The reasons underlying this rule seem clear. It is assumed that in most cases a conviction will do irreversible harm to an individual by damaging his reputation in the eyes of his fellows. The individual is seen as weak and defenseless, relative to society, and therefore in no position to sustain the consequences of an erroneous decision. An erroneous acquittal, on the other hand, damages society. If an individual who has actually committed a crime is not punished, he may commit the crime again, or more important, the deterrent effect of punishment for the violation of this crime may be diminished for others. Although these are serious outcomes, they are generally thought not to be so serious as the consequences of erroneous conviction for the innocent individual, since society is able to sustain an indefinite number of such errors without serious consequences. For these and perhaps other reasons, the decision rule to assume innocence exerts a powerful influence on legal proceedings.

TYPE 1 AND TYPE 2 ERRORS

Deciding on guilt or innocence is a special case of a problem to which statisticians have given considerable attention: the testing of hypotheses. Since most scientific work is done with samples, statisticians have developed techniques to guard against results which are due to chance sampling fluctuations. The problem, however, is that one may reject a finding that was actually correct as due to sampling fluctuations. There are, therefore, two kinds of errors: rejecting a hypothesis that is true and accepting one that is false. Usually the hypothesis is stated so that the former error (rejecting a hypothesis which is true) is the error that is thought to be the more important to avoid. This type of error is called an "error of the first kind," or a Type 1 error. The latter error (accepting a hypothesis which is false) is the less important error to avoid and is called an "error of the second kind," or a Type 2 error (Neyman, 1950:265–266).

To guard against chance fluctuations in sampling, statisticians test the probability that findings could have arisen by chance. At some predetermined probability (called the "alpha level"), usually 0.05 or less, the possibility that the findings arose by chance is rejected. This level means that there are 5 chances in 100 that one will reject a hypothesis which is true. Although these five chances indicate a real risk of error, it is not common to set the level much lower (say 0.001) because this raises the probability of making an error of the second kind.

A similar dilemma faces the judge or jury in deciding whether to convict or acquit in the face of uncertainty. Particularly in the adversary system of law, where professional attorneys seek to advance their arguments and refute those of their opponents, there is often considerable uncertainty even as to the facts of the case, let alone intangibles like intent. The maxim, "Better a thousand guilty men go free, than one innocent man be convicted," would mean, if taken literally rather than as a rhetorical flourish, that the alpha level for legal decisions is set quite low.

Although the legal decision rule is not expressed in so precise a form as a statistical decision rule, it represents a very similar procedure for dealing with uncertainty. There is one respect, however, in which it is quite different. Statistical decision procedures are recognized by those who use them as mere conveniences which can be varied according to the circumstances. The legal decision rule, in contrast, is an inflexible and binding moral rule which carries with it the force of long sanction and tradition. The assumption of innocence is a part of the social institution of law in Western society; it is explicitly stated in legal codes and is accepted as legitimate by jurists and usually by the general populace with only occasional grumbling, (e.g., a criminal is seen as "getting off" because of "legal technicalities").

DECISION RULES IN MEDICINE

Although the analogous rule for decisions in medicine is not so explicitly stated as the rule in law and probably is considerably less rigid, it would seem that there is such a rule in medicine which is as imperative in its operation as its analogue in law. Do physicians and the general public consider that rejecting the hypothesis of illness when it is true, or accepting it when it is false, is the error that is most important to avoid? It seems fairly clear that the rule in medicine may be stated as: "When in doubt, continue to suspect illness." That is, for a physician to dismiss a patient when he is actually ill is a Type 1 error, and to retain a patient when he is not ill is a Type 2 error.

Most physicians learn early in their training that it is far more culpable to dismiss a sick patient than to retain a well one. This rule is so pervasive and fundamental that it goes unstated in textbooks on diagnosis. It is occasionally mentioned explicitly in other contexts, however. Neyman (1950), for example, in his discussion of X-ray screening for tuberculosis states:

> [If the patient is actually well, but the hypothesis that he is sick is accepted, a Type 2 error] then the patient will suffer some unjustified anxiety and, perhaps, will be put to some unnecessary expense until further studies of his health will establish that any alarm about the state of his chest is unfounded. Also, the unjustified precautions ordered by the clinic may somewhat affect its reputation. On the other hand, should the hypothesis [of sickness] be true and yet the accepted hypothesis be [that he is well, a Type 1 error], then the patient will be in danger of losing the precious opportunity of treating the incipient disease in its beginning stages when the cure is not so difficult. Furthermore, the oversight by the clinic's specialist of the dangerous condition would affect the clinic's reputation even more than the unnecessary alarm. From this point of view, it appears that the error of rejecting the hypothesis [of sickness] when it is true is *far more important* to avoid than the error of accepting the hypothesis (of illness) when it is false [p. 270; italics added].

Although this particular discussion pertains to tuberculosis, it is pertinent to many other diseases also. From casual conversations with physicians, the impression one gains is that this moral lesson is deeply ingrained in the physician's personal code.

It is not only physicians who feel this way, however. This rule is grounded both in legal proceedings and in popular sentiment. Although there is some sentiment against Type 2 errors (unnecessary surgery, for instance), it has nothing like the force and urgency of the sentiment against Type 1 errors. A physician who dismisses a patient who subsequently dies of a disease that should have been detected is subject not only to legal action for negligence and possible loss of license for incompetence, but also to moral condemnation from his colleagues and from his own conscience for his delinquency. Nothing remotely resembling this amount of moral and legal suasion is brought to bear for committing a Type 2 error. Indeed, this error is sometimes seen as sound clinical practice, indicating a healthily conservative approach to medicine.

The discussion to this point suggests that physicians follow a decision rule which may be stated, "When in doubt, diagnose illness." If physicians are actually influenced by this rule, then studies of the validity of diagnosis should demonstrate the operation of the rule. That is, we should expect that objective studies of diagnostic errors should show that Type 1 and Type 2 errors do not occur with equal frequency, but in fact, that Type 2 errors far outnumber Type 1 errors. Unfortunately for our purposes, however, there are apparently only a few studies which provide the type of data which would adequately test the hypothesis. Although studies of the reliability of diagnosis abound (Garland, 1959) showing that physicians disagree with each other in their diagnoses of the same patients, these studies do not report the validity of diagnosis or the types of error which are made, with the following exceptions.

We can infer that Type 2 errors outnumber Type 1 errors from Bakwin's (1945) study of physicians' judgments regarding the advisability of tonsillectomy for 1000 school children.

> Of these, some 611 had had their tonsils removed. The remaining 389 were then examined by other physicians, and 174 were selected for tonsillectomy. This left 215 children whose tonsils were apparently normal. Another group of doctors was put to work examining these 215 children, and 99 of them were adjudged in need of tonsillectomy. Still another group of doctors was then employed to examine the remaining children, and nearly one-half were recommended for operation [p. 691–697].

Almost half of each group of children were judged to be in need of the operation. Even assuming that a small proportion of children needing tonsillectomy were missed in each examination (Type 1 error), the number of Type 2 errors in this study far exceeded the number of Type 1 errors.

In the field of roentgenology, studies of diagnostic error are apparently more highly developed than in other areas of medicine. Garland (1959:31) summarizes these findings, reporting that in a study of 14,867 films for tuberculosis signs, there were 1216 positive readings that turned out to be clinically negative (Type 2 error) and only 24 negative readings which turned out to be clinically active (Type 1 error)! This ratio (about 50:1) is apparently a fairly typical finding in roentgenographic studies. Since physicians are well aware of the provisional nature of radiological findings, this great discrepancy between the frequency of the types of error in film screening is not too alarming. On the other hand, it does provide objective evidence of the operation of the decision rule, "Better safe than sorry."

BASIC ASSUMPTIONS

The logic of this decision rule rests on two assumptions: First, disease is usually a determinate, inevitably unfolding process, which, if undetected and untreated, will grow to a point where it endangers the life or limb of the individual and, in the case of contagious diseases, the lives of others. This is not to say, of course, that physicians think of all diseases as determinate: Witness the concept of the "benign" condition. The point here is that the imagery of disease that the physician uses in attempting to reach a decision, his working hypothesis, is *usually* based on the deterministic model of disease.

Second, medical diagnosis of illness, unlike legal judgment, is not an irreversible act which does untold damage to the status and reputation of the patient. A physician may search for illness for an indefinitely long time, causing inconvenience for the patient, perhaps, but in the typical case, doing the patient no irradicable harm. Obviously, again, physicians do not always make this assumption. A physician who suspects epilepsy in a truck driver knows full well that his patient will probably never drive a truck again if the diagnosis is made, and the physician will go to great lengths to avoid a Type 2 error in this situation. Similarly, if a physician suspects that a particular patient has hypochondriacal trends, the physician will lean in the direction of a Type 1 error in a situation of uncertainty. These and other similar situations are exceptions, however. The physician's *usual* working assumption is that medical observation and diagnosis, in itself, is neutral and innocuous relative to the dangers resulting from disease.[2]

In the light of these two assumptions, therefore, it is seen as far better for the physician to chance a Type 2 error than a Type 1 error. These two assumptions will be examined and criticized in the remainder of the chapter. The assumption that Type 2 errors are relatively harmless will be considered first.

In recent discussions, it is increasingly recognized that in one area of medicine, psychiatry, the assumption that medical diagnosis can cause no irreversible harm to the patient's status is dubious. Psychiatric treatment, in many segments of the population and for many occupations, raises a question about the person's social status. It could be argued that in making a medical diagnosis the psychiatrist comes very close to making a legal decision, with its ensuing consequences for the person's reputation. One may argue that the Type 2 error in psychiatry, of judging a well person sick, is at least as much to be avoided as the Type 1 error, of judging the sick person well. Yet the psychiatrist's moral orientation, since he is first and foremost a physician, is guided by the medical, rather than the legal, decision rule. The psychiatrist continues to be more willing to err on the conservative side, to diagnose as ill when the person is healthy, even though it is no longer clear that this error is any more desirable than its opposite.

There is a more fundamental question about this decision rule, however, which concerns both physical illness and mental disorder. This question primarily concerns the first assumption: that disease is a determinate process. It also implicates the second assumption: that medical treatment does not have irreversible effects.

In recent years, physicians and social scientists have reported finding disease signs and deviant behavior prevalent in normal, noninstitutionalized populations. It has been shown, for instance, that deviant acts, some of a serious nature, are widely admitted by persons in random samples of normal populations (Wallerstein and Wyle, 1947; Porterfield, 1946; Kinsey, Pomeroy, and Martin, 1948). There is some evidence that suggests that grossly deviant, "psychotic" behavior

---

[2]Even though this assumption is widely held, it has been vigorously criticized within the medical profession. See, for example, Darley (1959). For a witty criticism of both assumptions, see Ratner (1962).

has at least temporarily existed in relatively large proportions of a normal population (Plunkett and Gordon, 1961; Clausen and Yarrow, 1955). Finally, there is a growing body of evidence that many signs of physical disease are distributed quite widely in normal populations. A survey of simple high blood pressure indicated that the prevalence ranged from 11.4 to 37.2% in the various subgroups studied (Rautaharju, Korvonen, and Keys, 1961).[3]

As stated in Chapter 3, physical defects and "psychiatric" deviancy exist in an uncrystallized form in large segments of the population. Lemert (1951) calls this type of behavior, which is often transitory, *primary deviation*. In his discussion of the doctor–patient relationship, Balint (1957) speaks of similar behavior as the "unorganized phase of illness" Balint seems to take for granted, however, that patients will eventually "settle down" to an "organized" illness. Yet it is possible that other outcomes may occur. A person in this stage may change jobs or wives instead, or merely continue in the primary deviation state indefinitely, without getting better or worse.

This discussion suggests that in order to estimate the probability that a person with a disease sign would become incapacitated because of the development of disease, investigations quite unlike existing studies would need to be conducted. These would be longitudinal studies in a random sample of a normal population, of outcomes in persons having signs of diseases in which no attempt was made to arrest the disease. It is true that there are a number of longitudinal studies in which the effects of treatment are compared with the effects of nontreatment. These studies, however, have always been conducted with clinical groups rather than with persons with disease signs who were located in field studies.[4] Even clinical trials appear to offer many difficulties, both from the ethical and scientific points of view (Hill, 1960). These difficulties would be increased many times in controlled field trials, as would the problems which concern the amount of time and money necessary. Without such studies, nevertheless, the meaning of many common disease signs remains somewhat equivocal.

Given the relatively small amount of knowledge about the distributions and natural outcomes of many diseases, it is possible that our conceptions of the danger of disease are exaggerated. To mention again the dramatic example cited earlier, until the late 1940s, histoplasmosis was thought to be a rare tropical disease with a uniform fatal outcome. Recently, however, it was discovered that it is widely prevalent and with fatal outcome or impairment extremely rare (Schwartz and Baum, 1957). It is conceivable that other diseases, such as some types of heart disease and mental disorder, may prove to be similar in character. Although no actuarial studies have been made which would yield the true probabilities of impairment, physicians usually set the Type 1 level quite high because they believe that the probability of impairment from making a Type 2 error is quite low. Let us now examine that assumption.

[3]Cf. Stokes and Dawber (1959); Dunn and Etter (1962).

[4]The Framingham Study is an exception to this statement. Even in this study, however, experimental procedures (random assignment to treatment and non treatment groups) were not used. Dawber, Moore and Mann (1957).

THE "SICK ROLE"

If, as has been argued here, much illness goes unattended without serious consequences, the assumption that medical diagnosis has no irreversible effects on the patients seems questionable.

> The patient's attitude to his illness is usually considerably changed during, and by, the series of physical examinations. These changes, which may profoundly influence the course of a chronic illness, are not taken seriously by the medical profession and, though occasionally mentioned, they have never been the subject of a proper scientific investigation [Balint, 1957:43].

There are grounds for believing that persons who avail themselves of professional services are under considerable strain and tension (if the problem could have been easily solved, they would probably have used more informal means of handling it). Social–psychological principles indicate that persons under strain are highly suggestible, particularly to suggestions from a prestigeful source, such as a physician.

It can be argued that the Type 2 error involves the danger of having a person enter the "sick role" (Parsons, 1950) in circumstances where no serious result would ensue if the illness were unattended. Perhaps the combination of a physician determined to find disease *signs*, if they are to be found, and the suggestible patient, searching for subjective *symptoms* among the many amorphous and usually unattended bodily impulses, is often sufficient to unearth a disease which changes the patient's status from that of well to sick and may also have effect on his familial and occupational status. [In Lemert's (1951) terms, the illness would be *secondary deviation* after the person has entered the sick role.]

There is a considerable body of evidence in the medical literature concerning the process in which the physician unnecessarily causes the patient to enter the sick role. Thus, in a discussion of "iatrogenic" (physician-induced) heart disease, this point is made:

> The physician, by calling attention to a murmur or some cardiovascular abnormality, even though functionally insignificant, may precipitate [symptoms of heart disease]. The experience of the work classification units of cardiac-in-industry programs, where patients with cardiovascular disease are evaluated as to work capacity, gives impressive evidence regarding the high incidence of such functional manifestations in persons with the diagnosis of cardiac lesion. [Warren and Wolter, 1954:77–84].

Although there is a tendency in medicine to dismiss this process as due to quirks of particular patients (e.g., as malingering, hypochondriasis, or as "merely functional disease," that is, functional for the patient), causation probably lies not in the patient but in medical procedures. Most people, perhaps, if they actually have the disease signs and are told by an authority, the physician, that they are ill, will obligingly come up with appropriate symptoms. A case history will illustrate this process. Under the heading ''It may be well to let sleeping dogs lie,'' a physician recounts the following case:

> Here is a woman, aged 40 years, who is admitted with symptoms of congestive cardiac failure, valvular disease, mitral stenosis and auricular fibrillation. She tells us that she did not know that there was anything wrong with her heart and that she had had no symptoms up to 5 years ago when her chest was x-rayed in the course of a mass radiography examination for tuberculosis. She was not suspected and this was only done in the course of routine at the factory. Her lungs were pronounced clear but she was told the she had an enlarged heart and was advised to go to a hospital for investigation and treatment. From that time she began to suffer from symptoms—breathlessness on exertion—and has been in the hospital 4 or 5 times since. Now she is here with congestive heart failure. She cannot understand why, from the time that her enlarged heart was discovered, she began to get symptoms [Gardiner-Hill, 1958:158].

What makes this kind of ''role-taking'' extremely important is that it can occur even when the diagnostic label is kept from the patient. By the way he is handled, the patient can usually infer the nature of the diagnosis, since in his uncertainty and anxiety he is extremely sensitive to subtleties in the physician's behavior. An example of this process (already cited in Chapter 3) is found in reports on treatment of battle fatigue. Speaking of psychiatric patients in the Sicilian campaign during World War II, a psychiatrist notes:

> Although patients were received at this hospital within 24 to 48 hours after their breakdown, a disappointing number, approximately 15 per cent, were salvaged for combat duty . . . any therapy, including usual interview methods that sought to uncover basic emotional conflicts or attempted to relate current behavior and symptoms with past personality patterns seemingly provided patients with logical reasons for their combat failure. The insights obtained by even such mild depth therapy readily convinced the patient and often his therapist that the limit of combat endurance had been reached as proved by vulnerable personality traits. Patients were obligingly cooperative in supplying details of their neurotic childhood, previous emotional difficulties, lack of aggressiveness and other dependence traits [Glass, 1953].

Glass goes on to say that removal of the soldier from his unit for treatment of any kind usually resulted in long-term neurosis. In contrast, if the soldier were given only superficial psychiatric attention and *kept with his unit*, chronic impairment was usually avoided. The implication is that removal from the military unit and psychiatric treatment symbolizes to the soldier, behaviorally rather than with verbal labels, the ''fact'' that he is a mental case.

The traditional way of interpreting these reactions of the soldiers, and perhaps the civilian cases, is in terms of malingering or feigning illness. The process of taking roles, however, as it is conceived of here, is not completely or even largely voluntary. (For a sophisticated discussion of role-playing, see Goffman [1959:17–21].) Vaguely defined impulses become ''real'' to the participants when they are organized under any one of a number of more or less interchangeable social roles. It can be argued that when a person is in a confused and suggestible state, when he organizes his feelings and behavior by using the sick role, and when his choice of roles is validated by a physician or others, he is "hooked" and will proceed on a career of chronic illness.[5]

IMPLICATIONS FOR RESEARCH

The hypothesis suggested by the preceding discussion is that physicians and the public typically overvalue medical treatment relative to nontreatment as a course of action in the face of uncertainty, and this overvaluation results in the creation as well as the prevention of impairment. This hypothesis, since it is based on scattered observations, is presented only to point out several areas where systematic research is needed.

From the point of view of assessing the effectiveness of medical practice, this hypothesis is probably too general to be used directly. Needed for such a task are hypotheses concerning the conditions under which error is likely to occur, the type of error that is likely, and the consequences of each type of error. Significant dimensions of the amount and type of error and its consequences would appear to be characteristics of the disease, the physician, the patient, and the organizational setting in which diagnosis takes place. Thus, for diseases such as pneumonia, which produce almost certain impairment unless attended and for which a quick and highly effective cure is available, the hypothesis is probably largely irrelevant. On the other hand, the hypothesis may be of considerable importance for diseases which have a less certain outcome and for which existing treatments are protracted and of uncertain value. Mental disorders and some types of heart disease are cases in point.

The working philosophy of the physician is probably relevant to the predominant type of errors made. Physicians who generally favor active intervention probably make more Type 2 errors than physicians who view their treatments only as assistance for natural bodily reactions to disease. The physician's perception of the personality of the patient may also be relevant; Type 2 errors are less likely if the physician defines the patient as a "crock," a person overly sensitive to discomfort, rather than as a person who ignores or denies disease.

Finally, the organizational setting is relevant to the extent that it influences the relationship between the doctor and the patient. In some contexts, as in medical practice in organizations such as the military or industrial setting, the physician is not so likely to feel personal responsibility for the patient as he would in other contexts, such as private practice. This may be due in part to the conditions of financial remuneration and, perhaps equally important, the sheer volume of patients dependent on the doctor's time. Cultural or class differences may also affect the amount of social distance between doctor and patient and therefore the amount of responsibility which the doctor feels for the patient. Whatever the

[5]Some of the findings of the Purdue Farm Cardiac Project support the position taken in this chapter. It was found, for example, that "iatrogenics" took more health precautions than "hidden cardiacs," suggesting that entry into the sick role can cause more social incapacity than the actual disease does. See Eichorn and Anderson (1962).

sources, the more the physician feels personally responsible for the patient, the more likely he is to make a Type 2 error.

To the extent that future research can indicate the conditions which influence the amount, type, and consequences of error, such research can make direct contributions to medical practice. Three types of research seem necessary in order to establish the true risks of impairment associated with common disease signs. First, controlled field trials of treated and untreated outcomes in a normal population would be needed. Second, perhaps in conjunction with these field trials, experimental studies of the effect of suggestion of illness by physicians and others would be necessary to determine the risks of unnecessary entry into the sick role.

Finally, studies of a mathematical nature seem to be called for. Suppose that physicians were provided with the results of the studies suggested here. How could these findings be introduced into medical practice as a corrective to cultural and professional biases in decision-making procedures? One promising approach is the strategy of evaluating the relative utility of alternative courses of action based upon decision theory or game theory (Chernoff and Moses, 1959).

Ledley and Lusted (1959) reviewed a number of mathematical techniques that may be applicable to medical decision making, one of these techniques being the use of the "expected value" equation, which is derived from game theory. Although their discussion pertains to the relative value of two treatment procedures, it is also relevant, with only slight changes in wording, to determining the expected values of treatment relative to nontreatment. The expected values of two treatments, they say, may be calculated from a simple expression involving only two kinds of terms: The probability that the diagnosis is correct and the absolute value of the treatment (at its simplest, the absolute value is the rate of cure for persons known to have the disease).

The "expected value" of a treatment is:

$$E_t = p_s v_s^s + (1 - p_s) v_h^s$$

(The superscript refers to the way the patient is treated, the subscript refers to his actual conditions; s signifies sick, h, healthy). That is, the expected value of a treatment is the probability p that the patient has the disease, multiplied by the value of the treatment for patients who actually have the disease, plus the probability that the patient does not have the disease $(1 - p)$, multiplied by the value (or "cost") of the treatment for patients who do not have the disease.

Similarly, the expected value of nontreatment is:

$$E_n = p_s v_s^h + (1 + p_s) v_h^h$$

That is, the expected value of nontreatment is the probability that the patient has the disease multiplied by the value (or "cost") of treating a person as healthy who is actually sick, plus the probability that the patient does not have the disease, multiplied by the value of not treating a healthy person.

The best course of action is indicated by comparing the magnitude of E_t and

E_n. If E_t is larger, treatment is indicated. If E_n is larger, nontreatment is indicated. Evaluating these equations involves estimating the probability of correct diagnosis and constructing a payoff matrix for the values of v_s^s (proportion of patients who actually had the disease who were cured by the treatment), v_h^s (the cost of treating a healthy person as sick: inconvenience, working days lost, surgical risks, unnecessary entry into sick role), v_s^h (cost of treating a sick person as well: a question involving the proportions of persons who spontaneously recover and the seriousness of results when the disease goes unchecked), and finally, v_h^h (the value of not treating a healthy person: medical expenses saved, working days, etc.).

To illustrate the use of the equation, Ledley and Lusted assign *arbitrary* absolute values in a case because, as they say: "The decision of value problems frequently involves intangibles such as moral and ethical standards which must, in the last analysis, be left to the physician's judgment" [p. 16]. One may argue, however, that it is better to develop a technique for systematically determining the absolute values of treatment and nontreatment, crude though the technique may be, than to leave the problem to the perhaps refined, but nevertheless obscure, judgment processes of the physician. Particularly in a matter of comparing the value of treatment and nontreatment, the problem is to avoid biases in the physician's judgment due to the kind of moral orientation discussed previously.

It is possible, moreover, that the difficulty met by Ledley and Lusted is not that the factors to be evaluated are "intangibles," but that they are expressed in seemingly incommensurate units. How does one weigh the risk of death against the monetary cost of treatment? How does one weigh the risk of physical or social disability against the risk of death? Although these are difficult questions to answer, the idea of leaving them to the physician's judgment is probably not conducive to an understanding of the problem.

Following the lead of the economists in their studies of utility, it may be feasible to reduce the various factors to be weighed to a common unit. How could the benefits, costs, and risks of alternative acts in medical practice be expressed in monetary units? One solution may be to use payment rates in disability and life insurance, which offer a comparative evaluation of the "cost" of death and permanent and temporary disability of various degrees. Although this approach does not include everything which physicians weigh in reaching decisions (pain and suffering cannot be weighed in this framework), it does include many of the major factors. It therefore would provide the opportunity of constructing a fairly realistic payoff matrix of absolute values, which would then allow for the determination of the relative value of treatment and nontreatment using the expected value equation.

Gathering data for the payoff matrix may make it possible to explore an otherwise almost inaccessible problem: the sometimes subtle conflicts of interest between the physician and the patient. Although it is fairly clear that medical intervention is unnecessary in particular cases, and that it is probably done for financial gain (Trussel, Ehrlich, and Morehead, 1962), the evaluation of the influence of remuneration on diagnosis and treatment is probably in most cases a fairly intricate matter, requiring precise techniques of investigation. If the payoff were calculated in terms of values to the patient *and* values to the physician, such problems could be explored. Less tangible values such as convenience and work satisfactions could be introduced into the matrix. The following statements by psychiatrists were taken from Hollingshead and Redlich's (1958) study of social class and mental disorder: "Seeing him every morning was a chore; I had to put him on my back and carry him for an hour." "He had to get attention in large doses, and this was hard to do." "The patient was not interesting or attractive; I had to repeat, repeat, repeat." "She was a poor unhappy, miserable woman—we were worlds apart [p. 344]."

This study strongly suggests that psychiatric diagnosis and treatment are influenced by the payoff for the psychiatrist as well as for the patient. In any type of medical decision, the use of the expected value equation may show the extent of the conflict of interest between the physician and patient and thereby shed light on the complex process of medical decision making.

Two Studies
of the Societal Reaction

6

THE case for making the societal reaction to rule-breaking a major independent variable in studies of deviant behavior has been succinctly stated by Kitsuse (1962):

> A sociological theory of deviance must focus specifically upon the interactions which not only define behaviors as deviant but also organize and activate the application of sanctions by individuals, groups, or agencies. For in modern society, the socially significant differentiation of deviants from the nondeviant populations is increasingly contingent upon circumstances of situation, place, social and personal biography, and the bureaucratically organized activities of agencies of control [p. 247–256].

In the case of mental disorder, psychiatric diagnosis is one of the crucial steps which "organizes and activates" the societal reaction, since the state is legally empowered to segregate and isolate those persons whom psychiatrists find to be committable because of mental illness.

It has been argued here, however, that mental illness may be more usefully considered to be a social status than a disease, since the symptoms of mental illness are vaguely defined and widely distributed, and the definition of behavior as symptomatic of mental illness is usually dependent upon social rather than medical contingencies. Furthermore, the argument continues, the status of the mental patient is more often an ascribed status, with conditions for status entry and exit external to the patient, than an achieved status with conditions for status entry dependent upon the patient's own behavior. According to this argument, the societal reaction is a fundamentally important variable in all stages of a deviant career.

The actual usefulness of a theory of mental disorder based on the societal reaction is largely an empirical question: To what extent is entry to and exit from the status of mental patient independent of the behavior or ''condition'' of the patient? This chapter explores this question for two phases of the societal reaction: the legal and psychiatric screening of persons alleged to be mentally ill and the decision to release patients resident in mental hospitals. These steps represent two of the official phases of the societal reaction, which occur after the alleged deviance has been called to the attention of the community. This chapter makes no reference to the initial rule-breaking or other situations which resulted in complaints or to the behavior of patients after release, but deals entirely with official decision procedures.

The purpose of the description that follows is to determine the extent of uncertainty that exists concerning patients' ''qualifications'' for involuntary confinement in a mental hospital and organizational reactions to this type of uncertainty. The data presented here indicate that, in the face of uncertainty, there is a strong presumption of illness by the court and the psychiatrists.[1] In the discussion that follows the presentation of findings, some of the causes, consequences, and implications of the presumption of illness are suggested.

LEGAL AND PSYCHIATRIC SCREENING OF INCOMING PATIENTS

The data upon which this phase of the study is based were drawn from psychiatrists' ratings of a sample of patients newly admitted to the public mental hospitals in a Midwestern state, official court records, interviews with court officials and psychiatrists, and our observations of psychiatric examinations in four courts.[2] The psychiatrists' ratings of new patients is considered first.

In order to obtain a rough measure of the incoming patient's qualifications for involuntary confinement, a survey of newly admitted patients was conducted with the cooperation of the hospital psychiatrists. All psychiatrists who made admission examinations in the three large mental hospitals in the state filled out a questionnaire for the first 10 consecutive patients they examined in the month of June 1962. A total of 223 questionnaires were returned by the 25 admission psychiatrists. Although these returns do not constitute a probability sample of all new patients admitted during the year, there were no obvious biases in the drawing of the sample. For this reason, this group of patients is considered typical of the newly admitted patients in Midwestern State.

The two principal legal grounds for involuntary confinement in the United States are the police power of the state (the state's right to protect itself from dangerous persons) and *parens patriae* (the State's right to assist those persons

---

[1]A general discussion of the presumption of illness is found in the first section of Chapter 5.

[2]This phase of the study was completed with the assistance of Daniel M. Culver.

who, because of their own incapacity, may not be able to assist themselves (Ross, 1959). As a measure of the first ground, the potential dangerousness of the patient, the questionnaire contained this item: "In your opinion, if this patient were released at the present time, is it likely he would harm himself or others?" The psychiatrists were given six options, ranging from Very Likely to Very Unlikely. Their responses were: Very Likely, 5%; Likely, 4%; Somewhat Likely, 14%; Somewhat Unlikely, 20%; Unlikely, 37%; Very Unlikely, 18%. (Three patients were not rated, 1%.)

As a measure of the second ground, *parens patriae*, the questionnaire contained the item: "Based on your observations of the patient's behavior, his present degree of mental impairment is: None . . . Minimal . . . Mild . . . Moderate . . . Severe. . . ." The psychiatrists' responses were: None, 2%; Minimal, 12%; Mild, 25%; Moderate, 42%; Severe, 17%. (Three patients were not rated, 1%.)

To be clearly qualified for involuntary confinement, a patient should be rated as likely to harm self or other (Very Likely, Likely, or Somewhat Likely) and / or as Severely Mentally Impaired. However, voluntary patients should be excluded from this analysis, since the court is not required to assess their qualifications for confinement. Excluding the 59 voluntary admissions (26% of the sample) leaves a sample of 164 involuntarily confined patients. Of these patients, 10 were rated as meeting both qualifications for involuntary confinement, 21 were rated as being severely mentally impaired but not dangerous, 28 were rated as dangerous but not severely mentally impaired, and 102 were rated as not dangerous nor as severely mentally impaired. (Three patients were not rated.)

According to these ratings, there is considerable uncertainty connected with the screening of newly admitted involuntary patients in the state, since a substantial majority (63%) of the patients did not clearly meet the statutory requirements for involuntary confinement. How does the agency responsible for assessing the qualifications for confinement, the court, react in the large numbers of cases involving uncertainty?

On the one hand, the legal rulings on this point by higher courts are quite clear. They have repeatedly held that there should be a presumption of sanity. If the burden of proof of insanity is to be on the petitioners, there must be a preponderance of evidence, and the evidence should be of a "clear and unexceptionable" nature.[3]

On the other hand, existing studies suggest that there is a presumption of illness by mental health officials. Mechanic (1962) describes admissions to two large mental hospitals located in an urban area in California:

> In the crowded state or county hospitals, which is the most typical situation, the psychiatrist does not have sufficient time to make a very complete psychiatric diagnosis, nor do his

---

[3]This is the typical phrasing in cases found under the heading, "Mental Illness," cited in *Decennial Legal Digest*.

psychiatric tools provide him with the equipment for an expeditious screening of the patient. . . .

In the two mental hospitals studied over a period of three months, the investigator never observed a case where the psychiatrist advised the patient that he did not need treatment. Rather, all persons who appeared at the hospital were absorbed into the patient population regardless of their ability to function adequately outside the hospital [p. 66–74]

A comment by Brown (1961:60[fn.]) suggests that it is a fairly general understanding among mental health workers that state mental hospitals in the United States accept all comers. In a study of 58 commitment proceedings, Miller (1966) found that some of the proceedings were "routine rituals."

Kutner (1962), describing commitment procedures in Chicago in 1962, also reports a strong presumption of illness by the staff of the Cook County Mental Health Clinic:

Certificates are signed as a matter of course by staff physicians after little or no examination. . . . The so-called examinations are made on an assembly-line basis, often being completed in two or three minutes, and never taking more than ten minutes. Although psychiatrists agree that it is practically impossible to determine a person's sanity on the basis of such a short and hurried interview, the doctors recommend confinement in 77 per cent of the cases. It appears in practice that the alleged-mentally-ill is presumed to be insane and bears the burden of proving his sanity in the few minutes allotted to him [p. 383–399].

These citations suggest that mental health officials handle uncertainty by presuming illness. Other investigators, however, have reported conflicting findings (Lowenthal, 1964; Mishler and Waxer, 1963).[4] To ascertain if the presumption of illness occurred in Midwestern State, intensive observations of screening procedures were conducted in the four courts with the largest volume of mental cases in the state. These courts were located in the two most populous cities in the state. Before giving the results of these observations, it is necessary to describe the steps in the legal procedures for hospitalization and commitment. The process of screening persons alleged to be mentally ill contain five steps in Midwestern State:

1. The application for judicial inquiry is made by three citizens. This application is heard by deputy clerks in two of the courts (C and D), by a court reporter in the third court, and by a court commissioner in the fourth court.
2. The intake examination is conducted by a hospital psychiatrist.
3. The psychiatric examination is conducted by two psychiatrists appointed by the court.

[4]Lowenthal found in her study that the patient's condition was the most important determinant of hospitalization. Mishler and Waxler report that 39% of applications to The Massachusetts Mental Health Center did not result in hospitalization, perhaps indicating that more rigorous screening was taking place.

4. There is an interview of the patient by the guardian *ad litem*, and a lawyer is appointed in three of the courts to represent the patient. (Court A did not use guardians *ad litem*.)
5. The judicial hearing is conducted by a judge.

These five steps take place roughly in the order listed, although in many cases (those cases designated as emergencies), Step 2, the intake examination, may occur before Step 1. Steps 1 and 2 usually take place on the same day or the day after hospitalization. Steps 3, 4, and 5 usually take place within a week of hospitalization. (In courts C and D, however, the judicial hearing is held only once a month.)

This series of steps would seem to provide ample opportunity for the presumption of health and a thorough assessment, therefore, of the patient's qualifications for involuntary confinement, since there are five separate points at which discharge could occur. According to our findings, however, these procedures usually do not serve the function of screening out persons who do not meet statutory requirements. At most of these decision points, in most of the courts, retention of the patient in the hospital was virtually automatic. A notable exception to this pattern was found in one of the three state hospitals; this hospital attempted to use Step 2, the intake examination, as a screening point to discharge patients whom the superintendent described as "illegitimate" (i.e., patients who do not qualify for involuntary confinement).[5] In the other two hospitals, however, this examination was perfunctory and virtually never resulted in a finding of health and a recommendation of discharge. In a similar manner, the other steps were largely ceremonial in character. For example, in court B, we observed 22 judicial hearings, all of which were conducted perfunctorily and with lightning rapidity. (The mean time of these hearings was 1.6 minutes.) The judge asked each patient two or three routine questions: "How do you feel?" "How are you being treated?" "Would you cooperate with the doctors if they think you should stay awhile?" *Whatever* the patient's answer, however, the judge immediately ended the hearing, managing in this way to average less than 2 minutes per patient. Even if the patient were extremely outspoken, no attempt was made to accommodate him. The following excerpt from an official transcript provides an example of such a case:

J. "How are you, Miss _____?
P. "Oh, pretty good."
J. "Are they treating you all right?"
P. "Yes."
J. "Any complaints?"

---

[5]Other exceptions occurred as follows: The deputy clerks in courts C and D appeared to exercise some discretion in turning away applications they considered improper or incomplete at Step 1; the judge in Court D appeared also to perform some screening at Step 5. For further description of these exceptions, see Scheff and Culver (1964).

P. "No. The only complaint I have is that they won't let me out."

J. "Well, do you want to get out?"

P. "Sure."

J. "What if the doctors say you should stay for a while to get well?

P. "Well, I don't see why I was sick, come in here in the first place."

J. "Well, let's see what the doctors say. Have they examined you yet—the doctors?"

P. "Well, examine me for what? For mental condition? I'm not mental as far as that is. The ones who brought me here—I think should be examined."

J. "Who brought you here?"

P. "The Police Department. Why, they come over to my house and they just grab people just like this. They try to make me say there is two tables when there is only one. What would you expect."

J. "All right, Miss _____."

P. "Where are your laws of today? I see that the laws are not very fair, not just either, or maybe your hospital needs money. We have to come here to help pay your bills. . . ." (The patient had become quite angry.)

J. "Well, we are overcrowded now."

P. "Well, then where is your justice in this world today? You have none, the way it looks to me. I think better justice should be done with your Police Department and your authority . . ."

J. "All right, Miss _____, thank you."

P. "That's all I ask you to do. There are probably many like me today are facing the same problems that I do and they are not even guilty to be put up in a mental institution . . ."

J. "All right."

It should be noted that the judge made no attempt to inform this voluble patient of her right to counsel, which might have relieved her considerably. In this court, informing the patient of her rights was supposedly done through the guardian *ad litem*. The patient, however, had no way of knowing this at the time of the hearing.

Our observations of the guardian's interviews suggested, furthermore, that the guardians were not likely to take the patients's side, since, like the examining psychiatrists, they were paid a flat fee for each case. That is, their rate of pay depended on the rapidity with which they could finish. In recommending hospitalization, they were avoiding interruption of the already occurring process of hospitalization and treatment; hence, their interview could be quite short. If, on the other hand, they wished to recommend discharge, they would have to interrupt an on-going process, take the responsibility for such interruption, and build a case for discharge. Building such a case would have required considerably more time, thus severely reducing their rate of pay.

In the 12 interviews we observed by guardians, none of the guardians informed the patient of his rights. This omission was especially striking in the three interviews of one guardian, since he was quite vocal about the rights of the patients when interviewed beforehand:

Q: "What is the function of the guardian *ad litem*?"

A: "To protect the legal rights of the ward."

Q: "What are these rights?"

A: "*One*: trial by jury.
   Two: right to his own attorney.
   Three: right to a hearing.
   Four: right to petition for a re-examination.
   I think that the right to private counsel is very important."

Noticing that in none of the three cases did he inform the patient of any of the rights he quoted, the interviewer asked him about the third case in which this information might have been particularly useful to the patient.

Q: "I don't remember for sure, but did you tell John _____ (the last patient interviewed) about his right to a lawyer? Was this an oversight or did you skip it purposely?"

A: "I didn't purposely skip it so that he wouldn't know about it but I was conscious of not telling him. You know lawyers don't work for nothing and I had it in the back of my mind that Mr. _____ (the patient) was not able to pay for any lawyer because, as you remember, he said he had enough to get to Minneapolis. A guy hates to refer a client when he knows that client can't pay."

What appeared to be the key role in justifying these procedures was played in Step 3, the examination by the court-appointed psychiatrists. In our informal discussions of screening with the judges and other court officials, these officials made it clear that although the statutes give the court the responsibility for the decision to confine or release persons alleged to be mentally ill, they would rarely, if ever, take the responsibility for releasing a mental patient without a medical recommendation to that effect. The crucial question, therefore, for the entire screening process is whether or not the court-appointed psychiatric examiners presume illness. The remainder of the chapter considers this question.

Our observations of 116 judicial hearings raised the question of the adequacy of the psychiatric examination. Eighty-six of the hearings failed to establish that the patients were "mentally ill" (according to the criteria stated by the judges in interviews).[6] Indeed, the behavior and responses of 48 of the patients at the hearings seemed completely unexceptionable. Yet the psychiatric examiners had not recommended the release of a single one of these patients. Examining the court records of 80 additional cases, we found still not a single recommendation for release.

Although the recommendation for treatment of 196 out of 196 consecutive cases strongly suggests that the psychiatric examiners were presuming illness, particularly when we observed 48 of these patients to be responding appropriately, it is conceivable that this is not the case. The observer for this study was not a psychiatrist (he was a first-year graduate student in social work), and it is possible that he could have missed evidence of disorder that a psychiatrist might have

---

[6]In interviews with the judges, the following criteria were named: appropriateness of behavior and speech, understanding of the situation, and orientation.

seen. It was therefore arranged for the observer to be present at a series of psychiatric examinations in order to determine whether the examinations appeared to be merely formalities or whether, on the other hand, through careful examination and interrogation, the psychiatrists were able to establish illness even in patients whose appearance and responses were not obviously disordered. The observer was instructed to note the examiner's procedures, the criteria they appeared to use in arriving at their decision, and their reaction to uncertainty.

Each of the courts discussed here employs the services of a panel of physicians as medical examiners. The physicians are paid a flat fee of $10 per examination and are usually assigned from 3 to 5 patients for each trip to the hospital. In court A, most of the examinations are performed by two psychiatrists, who go to the hospital once a week, seeing from 5 to 10 patients a trip. In court B, C, and D, a panel of local physicians is used. These courts seek to arrange the examinations so that one of the examiners is a psychiatrist, the other a general practitioner. Court B has a list of four such pairs and appoints each pair for a month at a time. Courts C and D have a similar list, apparently with some of the same names as court B.

To obtain physicians who were representative of the panel used in these courts, we arranged to observe the examinations of the two psychiatrists employed by the court A and one of the four pairs of physicians used in court B, one a psychiatrist, the other a general practitioner. We observed 13 examinations in court A and 13 examinations in court B. The judges in courts C and D refused to give us the names of the physicians on their panels, and we were unable to observe examinations in these courts. (The judge in court D stated that he did not want these physicians harassed in their work, since it was difficult to obtain their services even under the best of circumstances.) In addition to observing the examinations by four psychiatrists, we interviewed three other psychiatrists used by these courts.

The medical examiners followed two lines of questioning. One line was to inquire about the circumstances that led to the patient's hospitalization, the other was to ask standard questions to test the patient's orientation and his capacity for abstract thinking by asking him the date, the President, Governor, proverbs, and problems requiring arithmetic calculation. These questions were often asked very rapidly, and the patient was usually allowed only a very brief time to answer.

It should be noted that the psychiatrists in these courts had access to the patient's record (which usually contained the Application for Judicial Inquiry and the hospital chart notes on the patient's behavior), and that several of the psychiatrists stated that they almost always familiarized themselves with this record before making the examination. To the extent that they were familiar with the patient's circumstances from such outside information, it is possible that the psychiatrists were basing their diagnosis of illness less on the rapid and peremptory examination than on this other information. Although this was true to some extent, the importance of the record can easily be exaggerated, both because of the deficiencies in the typical record and because of the way it is usually utilized by the examiners.

The deficiencies of the typical record were easily discerned in the approximately 100 applications and hospital charts which the author read. Both the applications and charts were extremely brief and sometimes garbled. Moreover, in some of the cases where the author and interviewer were familiar with the circumstances involved in the hospitalization, it was not clear that the complainant's testimony was any more accurate than the version presented by the patient. Often the original complaint was so paraphrased and condensed that the application seemed to have little meaning.

The attitude of the examiners toward the record was such that even in those cases where the record was ample, it often did not figure prominently in their decision. Disparaging remarks about the quality and usefulness of the record were made by several of the psychiatrists. One of the examiners was apologetic about his use of the record, giving us the impression that he thought that a good psychiatrist would not need to resort to any information outside his own personal examination of the patient. A casual attitude toward the record was openly displayed in 6 of the 26 examinations we observed. In these 6 examinations, the psychiatrist could not (or in three cases, did not bother to) locate the record and conducted the examination without it, with one psychiatrist making it a point of pride that he could easily diagnose most cases "blind."

In his observations of the examinations, the interviewer was instructed to rate how well the patient responded by noting his behavior during the interview, whether he answered the orientation and concept questions correctly, and whether he denied and explained the allegations which resulted in his hospitalization. If the patient's behavior during the interview obviously departed from conventional social standards (e.g., in one case the patient refused to speak), if he answered the orientation questions incorrectly, or if he did not deny and explain the petitioners' allegations, the case was rated as meeting the statutory requirements, for hospitalization. Of the 26 examinations observed, 8 were rated as "Criteria Met."

If, on the other hand, the patient's behavior was appropriate, his answers correct, and he denied and explained the petitioners' allegations, the interviewer rated the case as not meeting the statutory criteria. Of the 26 cases, 7 were rated as "Criteria Not Met." Finally, if the examination was inconclusive, but the interviewer felt that more extensive investigation might have established that the criteria were met, he rated the cases as "Criteria Possibly Met." Of the 26 examined, 11 were rated in this way. The interviewer was instructed that whenever he was in doubt to avoid using the rating "Criteria Not Met."

Even giving the examiners the benefit of the doubt, the interviewer's ratings were that a substantial majority of the examinations he observed failed to establish that the statutory criteria were met. The relationship between the examiners' recommendations and the interviewer's ratings are shown in Table 6.1.

TABLE 6.1.   Observer's Ratings and Examiners' Recommendations

Examiners' recommendations	Observer's ratings			
	Criteria met	Criteria possibly met	Criteria not met	Total
Commitment	7	9	2	18
30-day observation	1	2	3	6
Release	0	0	2	2
Total	8	11	7	26

The interviewer's ratings suggest that the examinations established that the statutory criteria were met in only 8 cases, but the examiners recommended that the patient be retained in the hospital in 24 cases, leaving 16 cases that the interviewer rated as uncertain and in which retention was recommended by the examiners. The observer also rated the patient's expressed desires regarding staying in the hospital and the time taken by the examination. The ratings of the patient's desire concerning staying or leaving the hospital were: Leave, 14 cases; Indifferent, 1 case; Stay, 9 cases; and Not Ascertained, 2 cases. In only one of the 14 cases in which the patient wished to leave was the interviewer's rating Criteria Met.

Interviews ranged in length from 5 minutes to 17 minutes, with the mean time being 10.2 minutes. Most of the interviews were hurried, with the questions of the examiners coming so rapidly that the examiner often interrupted the patient or one examiner interrupted the other. All of the examiners seemed quite hurried. One psychiatrist, after stating in an interview (before we observed his examinations) that he usually took about 30 mintues, stated: "It's not remunerative. I'm taking a hell of a cut. I can't spend 45 minutes with a patient. I don't have the time, it doesn't pay." In the 8 examinations that we observed, this physician actually spent 8, 10, 5, 8, 8, 7, 17, and 11 minutes with the patients, or an average of 9.2 minutes.

In these short time periods, it is virtually impossible for the examiner to extend his investigation beyond the standard orientation questions and a short discussion of the circumstances which brought the patient to the hospital. In those cases where the patient answered the orientation questions correctly, behaved appropriately, and explained his presence at the hospital satisfactorily, the examiners did not attempt to assess the reliability of the petitioner's complaints or to probe further into the patient's answers. Given the fact that in most of these instances the examiners were faced with borderline cases, that they took little time in the examinations, and that they usually recommended commitment, we can only conclude that their decisions were based largely on a presumption of illness. Supplementary observations reported by the interviewer support this conclusion.

After each examination, the observer asked the examiner to explain the criteria he used in arriving at his decision. The observer also had access to the examiner's official report so that he could compare what the examiner said about the case with the record of what actually occurred during the interview. This supplementary information supports the conclusion that the examiner's decisions are based on the presumption of illness and sheds light on the manner in which these decisions are reached:

1. The "evidence' upon which the examiners based their decision to retain often seemed arbitrary.
2. In some cases, the decision to retain was made even when no evidence could be found.
3. Some of the psychiatrists' remarks suggest prejudgment of the cases.
4. Many of the examinations were characterized by carelessness and haste.

The first question, concerning the arbitrariness of the psychiatric evidence, is considered here. In the weighing of the patient's responses during the interview, the physician appeared not to give the patient credit for the large number of correct answers he gave. In the typical interview, the examiner may ask the patient 15 or 20 questions: the date, time, place, who is President, Governor, etc., what is $11 \times 10 \times 11 \times 11$, etc., explain "Don't put all your eggs in one basket," "A rolling stone gathers no moss," etc. The examiners appeared to feel that a wrong answer established lack of orientation, even when it was preceded by a series of correct answers. In other words, the examiners do not establish any standard score on the orientation questions, which would give an objective picture of the degree to which the patient answered the questions correctly, but seem at times to search until they find an incorrect answer.

For those questions that were answered incorrectly, it was not always clear whether the incorrect answers were due to the patient's "mental illness," the time pressure in the interview, the patient's lack of education, or other causes. Some of the questions used to establish orientation were sufficiently difficult that persons not mentally ill might have difficulty with them. One of the examiners always asked, in a rapid-fire manner: "What year is it?" What year was it 7 years ago? Seventeen years before that?" etc. Only two of the five patients who were asked this series of questions were able to answer it correctly. However, it is a moot question whether a higher percentage of persons in a household survey would be able to do any better. To my knowledge, none of the orientation questions that are used have been checked in a normal population.

Finally, the interpretations of some of the evidence as showing mental illness seemed capricious. Thus, one of the patients when asked, "In what ways are a banana, an orange, and an apple alike?" answered, "They are all something to eat." This answer was used by the examiner in explaining his recommendation to commit. The observer had noted that the patient's behavior and responses seemed appropriate and asked why the recommendation to commit had been made. The doctor stated that her behavior had been bizarre (possibly referring to her alleged promiscuity), her affect inappropriate (''When she talked about being pregnant, it was without feeling,''), and with regard to the question above: ''She wasn't able to say a banana and an orange were fruit. She couldn't take it one step further, she had to say it was something to eat.'' In other words, this psychiatrist was suggesting that in her thinking, the patient manifested ''concreteness,'' which is held to be a symptom of mental illness. Yet in her other answers to classification questions and to proverb interpretations, concreteness was not apparent, suggesting that the examiner's application of this test was arbitrary. In another case, the physician stated that he thought the patient was suspicious and distrustful because he had asked about the possibility of being represented by counsel at the judicial hearing. The observer felt that these and other similar interpretations may possibly be correct, but that further investigation of the supposedly incorrect responses would be needed to establish that they were manifestations of disorientation.

In several cases, where even this type of evidence was not available, the examiners still recommended retention in the hospital. Thus, one examiner employed by court A stated that he had recommended 30-day observation for a patient whom he had thought *not* to be mentally ill on the grounds that the patient, a young man, could not get along with his parents and ''might get into trouble.'' This examiner went on to say: ''We always take the conservative side (commitment or observation). Suppose a patient should commit suicide. We always make the conservative decision. I had rather play it safe. There's no harm in doing it that way.'' It appeared to the observer that ''playing safe'' meant that even in those cases where the examination established nothing, the psychiatrists did not consider recommending release. Thus in one case, the examination had established that the patient had a very good memory, was oriented, and spoke quietly and seriously. The observer recorded his discussion with the physician after the examination as follows:

> When the doctor told me he was recommending commitment for this patient too (he had also recommended commitment in the two examinations held earlier that day) he laughed because he could see what my next question was going to be. He said, ''I already recommended the release of two patients this month.'' This sounded like it was the maximum amount the way he said it.

Apparently, this examiner felt that he had a very limited quota on the number of patients he could recommend for release (less than 2% of those examined).

The language used by these physicians tends to intimate that mental illness was found even when reporting the opposite. Thus in one case, the recommendation stated: ''No gross evidence of delusions or hallucinations.'' This statement is misleading since not only was there no gross evidence, there was not any evidence, not even the slightest suggestion of delusions or hallucinations brought out by the interview.

These remarks suggest that the examiners prejudge the cases they examine. Several further comments indicate prejudgment. One physician stated that he thought that most crimes of violence were committed by patients released too early from mental hospitals. (This is an erroneous belief.[7]) He went on to say that he thought that all mental patients should be kept in the hospital at least 3 months, indicating prejudgment concerning his examinations. Another physician, after a very short interview (8 minutes), told the observer: "On the schizophrenics, I don't bother asking them more questions when I can see they're schizophrenic because *I know what they are going to say*. You could talk to them another half hour and not learn any more." Another physician, finally, contrasted cases in which the patient's family or others initiated hospitalization ("petition cases," the great majority of cases) with those cases initiated by the court: "The petition cases are pretty *automatic*. If the patient's own family wants to get rid of him you know there is something wrong."

The lack of care that characterized the examinations is evident in the forms on which the examiners make their recommendations. On most of these forms, whole sections have been left unanswered. Others are answered in a peremptory and uninformative way. For example, in the section entitled "Physical Examination," the question is asked: "Have you made a physical examination of the patient? State fully what is the present physical condition." A typical answer is "Yes. Fair.," or "Is apparently in good health." Since in none of the examinations we observed was the patient actually physically examined, these answers appear to be mere guesses. One of the examiners used regularly in court B, to the question "On what subject or in what way is derangement now manifested?" always wrote in "Is mentally ill." The omissions and the almost flippant brevity of these forms, together with the arbitrariness, lack of evidence, and prejudical character of the examinations, discussed previously all support the observer's conclusion that, except in very unusual cases, the psychiatric examiner's recommendation to retain the patient is virtually automatic.

Lest it be thought that these results are unique to a particularly backward Midwestern State, it should be pointed out that this state is noted for its progressive psychiatric practices. It will be recalled that a number of the psychiatrists employed by the court as examiners had finished their psychiatric residencies, which is not always the case in many other states. A still common practice in other states is to employ as members of the "Lunacy Panel" partially retired physicians with no psychiatric training whatever. This was the case in 1959 in Stockton, California, where I observed hundreds of hearings at which these physicians were present. It may be indicative of some of the larger issues underlying the question of civil commitment that, in these hearings, the physicians played very little part; the judge controlled the questioning of the relatives

[7]See Footnote to Table 4.1. or See Nunnally (1961).

and patients, and the hearings were often a model of impartial and thorough investigation.

Ratings of the qualifications for involuntary confinement of patients newly admitted to the public mental hospitals in a Midwestern state, together with observations of judicial hearings and psychiatric examinations by the observer connected with the present study, suggest that the decision as to the mental condition of a majority of the patients is an uncertain one. The fact that the courts seldom release patients and the perfunctory manner in which the legal and medical procedures are carried out suggest that the judicial decision to retain patients in the hospital for treatment is routine and largely based on the presumption of illness. Three reasons for this presumption are: financial, ideological, and political.

Our discussions with the examiners indicated that one reason that they perform biased "examinations" is that their rate of pay is a flat fee, not determined by the length of time spent with the patient. In recommending retention, the examiners are refraining from interrupting the hospitalization and commitment procedures already in progress and thereby allowing someone else, usually the hospital, to make the effective decision to release or commit. In order to recommend release, however, they would have to build a case showing why these procedures should be interrupted. Building such a case would take much more time than is presently expended by the examiners, thereby reducing their fee.

A more fundamental reason for the presumption of illness by the examiners, and perhaps the reason why this practice is allowed by the courts, is the interpretation of current psychiatric doctrine by the examiners and court officials. These officials make a number of assumptions, which are now thought to be of doubtful validity:

1. The condition of mentally ill persons deteriorates rapidly without psychiatric assistance.
2. Effective psychiatric treatments exist for most mental illnesses.
3. Unlike surgery, there are no risks involved in involuntary psychiatric treatment: It either helps or is neutral; it can't hurt.
4. Exposing a prospective mental patient to questioning, cross-examination, and other screening procedures exposes him to the unnecessary stigma of trial-like procedures and may do further damage to his mental condition.
5. There is an element of danger to self or others in most mental illness. It is better to risk unnecessary hospitalization than the harm the patient may do himself or others.

Many psychiatrists and others now argue that none of these assumptions is necessarily correct.

First, the assumption that psychiatric disorders usually get worse without treatment rests on very little other than evidence of an anecdotal character. There is just as much evidence that most acute psychological and emotional upsets are self-terminating.[8]

Second, it is still not clear, according to systematic studies evaluating psychotherapy, drugs, etc., that most psychiatric interventions are any more effective, on the average, than no treatment at all.[9]

Third, there is very good evidence that involuntary hospitalization and social isolation may affect the patient's life: his job, his family affairs, etc. There is some evidence that too hasty exposure to psychiatric treatment may convince the patient that he is "sick," prolonging what might have been an otherwise transitory episode.[10]

Fourth, this assumption is correct, as far as it goes. But it is misleading because it fails to consider what occurs when the patient who does not wish to be hospitalized is forcibly treated. Such patients often become extremely indignant and angry, particularly in the case, as often happens, when they are deceived into coming to the hospital on some pretext.

Fifth, the element of danger is usually exaggerated both in amount and degree. In the psychiatric survey of new patients in state mental hospitals, danger to self or others was mentioned in about a fourth of the cases. Furthermore, in those cases where danger is mentioned, it is not always clear that the risks involved are greater than those encountered in ordinary social life. This issue has been discussed by Ross (1959), an attorney:

> A truck driver with a mild neurosis who is "accident prone" is probably a greater danger to society than most psychotics; yet he will not be committed for treatment, even if he would be benefited. The community expects a certain amount of dangerous activity. I suspect that as a class, drinking drivers are a greater danger than the mentally ill, and yet the drivers are tolerated or punished with small fines rather than indeterminate imprisonment [p. 962].

From our observations of the medical examinations and other commitment procedures, we formed a very strong impression that the doctrines of danger to self or others, early treatment, and the avoidance of stigma were invoked partly because the officials believed them to be true and partly because they provided convenient justification for a preexisting policy of summary action, minimal investigation, avoidance of responsibility, and after the patient is in the hospital, indecisiveness and delay.

---

[8]For a review of epidemiological studies of mental disorder see Plunkett and Gordon (1960). Most of these studies suggest that at any given point in time, psychiatrists find a substantial proportion of persons in normal populations to be "mentally ill." One interpretation of this finding is that much of the deviance in these studies is self-limiting.

[9]For an assessment of the evidence regarding the effectiveness of electroshock, drugs, psychotherapy, and other psychiatric treatments, see Eysenck (1961). Author's note: my argument here is now (1984) outdated. There is new evidence that some psychoactive drugs and some psychotherapies are more effective than no treatment.

[10]For examples from military psychiatry, see Glass (1953) and Bushard (1957). For a discussion of essentially the same problem in the context of a civilian mental hospital. Cf. Erikson (1957).

The policy of presuming illness is probably both cause and effect of political pressure on the court from the community. The judge, an elected official runs the risk of being more heavily penalized for erroneously releasing than for erroneously retaining patients. Since the judge personally appoints the panel of psychiatrists to serve as examiners, he can easily transmit the community pressure to them by failing to reappoint a psychiatrist whose examinations were inconveniently thorough.

Some of the implications of these findings for the sociology of deviant behavior are briefly summarized. The foregoing discussion of the reasons that the psychiatrists tend to presume illness suggests that the motivations of the key decision makers in the screening process may be significant in determining the extent and direction of the societal reaction. In the case of psychiatric screening of persons alleged to be mentally ill, the social differentiation of the deviant from the nondeviant population appears to be materially affected by the financial ideological, and political position of the psychiatrists, who are, in this instance, the key agents of social control.

Under these circumstances, the character of the societal reaction appears to undergo a marked change from the pattern of normalization which occurs in the community. The official societal reaction appears to reverse the presumption of normality reported by the Cummings (1957:102) as a characteristic of informal societal reaction and instead exaggerates both the amount and degree of deviance. Thus, one extremely important contingency influencing the severity of the societal reaction may be whether or not the original rule-breaking comes to official notice. This chapter suggests that in the area of mental disorder, perhaps in contrast to other areas of deviant behavior, if the official societal reaction is invoked, for whatever reason, social differentiation of the deviant from the nondeviant population will usually occur.

This section has sought to demonstrate that the behavior or ''condition'' of the person alleged to be mentally ill is not usually an important factor in the decision of officials to retain or release new patients from the mental hospital. The marginal nature of the majority of the cases, the peremptoriness and inadequacy of most of the examinations, when considered in light of the fact that virtually every patient is recommended for commitment, would appear to demonstrate this proposition. Additional illustrative material was discussed which also supported this conclusion. The next section is a discussion of a study of the release of patients after they have been treated.

RELEASE OF PATIENTS: PSYCHIATRIC AND SOCIAL CONTINGENCIES

In this discussion, we seek to formulate questions concerning mental disorder in such a way that research and discussion in this area could be integrated into the general body of sociological theory. That is, we have considered the mental patient to be a person occupying a special status in the social structure. Viewed in this way, questions concerning the course of treated ''mental illness'' become problems of status mobility: diagnosis and cure become, sociologically, entry and exit to and from the status of a mental patient. Since a career may be viewed as the occupancy of a status over a period of time, questions concerning the conditions under which confinement in a mental hospital is initiated and terminated become questions of "career contingencies."

The contingency which is usually considered to be determinate in the mobility of mental patients is the psychiatric condition of the patient himself. The status of the mental patient, that is, is considered to be an achieved status, dependent only on the patient's behavior. We have argued, however, that the mental patient's status is partly ascribed. Lemert (1951:55–56) points to the putative character of the societal reaction, and Goffman (1961) states:

> The society's official view is that inmates of mental hospitals are there primarily because they are suffering from mental illness. However, in the degree that the "mentally ill" outside hospitals numerically approach or surpass those inside hospitals, one could say that mental patients distinctively suffer not from mental illness, but from contingencies [p. 135].

This passage suggests the hypothesis that contingencies external to the patient (such as the number of hospital beds available, the willingness of the community to accept a patient that the hospital wishes to discharge, etc.) may be as fateful for a patient's career as the hospital's evaluation of his medical and legal qualification for confinement.

The results of the numerous prior studies of the relationship between the social and psychiatric characteristics of patients and release do not appear to be useful in evaluating the hypothesis that social and situational characteristics may be crucial in release. These studies consistently show a relationship between social variables and release rates without, however, controlling for the patients' qualifications for release.[11] It is thus not clear, (using class as an example) whether lower-class patients have poorer chances for release because they are less qualified or because class, independently of qualifications, somehow determines release chances. This ambiguity, which runs like a thread through most of the literature on social medicine, is also characteristic of studies of the release of mental patients.

This section seeks to test the hypothesis that social contingencies may be crucial by examining the joint effect of social and psychiatric contingencies on release plans for mental patients in a Midwestern state. If mental patients "distinctively suffer not from mental illness, but from contingencies," we would expect to find that the decision to release or retain can be explained in terms of the patient's condition for only some of the patients, and that for the remainder,

---

[11]One such study (Linn, 1959) cites other representative studies (see p. 281, footnote 4). Two studies with a different approach but the same limitations are: Simmons, Davis, and Spencer (1956) and Freeman and Simmons (1961). The study by Dinitz, Lefton, Angrist, and Pasamanick (1961) is an exception to this statement; their results support the theory discussed here (see Dinitz *et al.*, Chapter 3, footnote 41).

contingencies such as type of hospital, the patient's age, and his length of confinement must be introduced.[12]

The data used in this study were obtained through standard questionnaires distributed to the staff of all public mental hospitals in a Midwestern state. On June 1,1962, a 4% systematic sample ($N = 555$) of patients was drawn from lists which comprised the entire patient population in the state, 13,684 persons at the time the sample was drawn. (Hospitals for the criminally insane and mentally retarded were not included.) Of the 555 questionnaires distributed, 4 were not returned, and 21 patients were checked as released (10), transferred (3), or died (8) during the period (about 2 weeks) between the drawings of the sample and the interviewing of the patients, leaving a total sample of 530 cases.

The hospital official legally responsible for the patient (a psychiatrist, social worker, or hospital superintendent) interviewed each patient whose name fell into the sample and filled out the questionnaire on the basis of the interview and other knowledge he had of the patient. A total of 63 officials participated in the study by returning these questionnaires. The questionnaire contained 24 questions about the patient's history and his present condition and included questions about the examiner's rating of the patient's degree of mental impairment, the likelihood the patient would harm himself or others if released, personal characteristics such as the patient's age, sex, education, usual occupation, etc., and whether or not the hospital was making plans for releasing the patient. Before discussing the relationship between release plans and contingencies, I give a brief description of the characteristics of the patients in the sample.

The ratings of the patient's education and usual occupation suggest that the hospital population is predominantly composed of persons of low social class: Only 15% of the patients in the sample had completed high school, and only a third of these had one or more years of college. Four percent of the patients had professional, managerial, or technical, usual occupations, and 5% clerical and sales occupations, the rest of the sample falling into manual and farm labor classification and non-labor-force. Twenty-eight percent of the patients were rated as being first admissions. A simple check of the proportion male in the sample against the proportion male in the total hospital population fails to show bias in the sampling and questionnaire collection: 50% of the patients in the sample were male, which is the same proportion reported in the total census by the Midwest State division of mental hospitals for the month in which the survey was conducted.

Release plans were reported for 43 of the patients (8% of the total sample). One important contingency that would be expected to influence the number of release plans is type of hospital. In Midwestern State, public mental hospitals may be classified into two categories: receiving hospitals, where most first admissions are brought, and transfer hospitals, whose patient populations are

---

[12]Of the social characteristics included in the questionnaire, these three were most strongly associated with release plans.

largely made up of persons transferred from the receiving hospitals. The receiving hospitals appear to be, on the whole, more treatment and release-oriented than the transfer hospitals. All three of the receiving hospitals maintained staffs of full-time psychiatrists, psychologists, and social workers. Most of the transfer hospitals, however, maintained only a single social worker or a part-time or consulting psychiatrist. The responses to one item on the questionnaire concerning treatment show, for example, that 27% of the patients in the transfer hospitals received no form of treatment whatever except "custodial care." In the receiving hospitals, only 15% of the patients were rated as receiving no treatment.

The amount of release planning in the receiving hospitals also exceeds that in the transfer hospitals, as shown in Table 6.2.

Table 6.2 indicates a substantial difference in the proportion of release plans between the two types of hospitals: 28% for the receiving hospitals but only 3% for the transfer hospitals. This difference could be interpreted to mean that patients in the transfer hospitals have considerably less chance for release than those in receiving hospitals simply because they happen to be in transfer hospitals. An alternative interpretation, however, is that the patients in the transfer hospitals are less qualified for release. Before making any interpretation, knowledge of the qualifications of each group of patients for release is necessary.

Two items on the questionnaire are relevant to the patients' qualifications for release. (The same items were used in the first study in this chapter, cf. p. 130.) The first item concerns the potential harm the patient may commit if released: "In your opinion, if this patient were released at the present time, is it likely that he would harm himself or others?" The examiner was allowed six options in answering, ranging from Very Likely to Very Unlikely. The responses to this question were as follows: Very Likely, 6%; Likely, 9.2%; Somewhat Likely, 12.2%; Somewhat Unlikely, 17.9%; Unlikely, 32.8%; Very Unlikely, 20.8%; (No rating, 0.6%).

The second item relevant to patients' qualifications for release concerned the degree of mental impairment: "Based on your observations of the patient's behavior, his present degree of mental impairment is: None, Minimal, Mild, Moderate, or Severe." The responses were 0.6%, 4.5%, 18.7%, 45.0%, and 30.8%, respectively, and .6% not rated.

These two ratings, taken together, may be used as a measure of the patient's

TABLE 6.2. Release Plans in Receiving and Transfer Hospitals

	Receiving	Transfer	Total
Release plans	31(28%)	12(3%)	43
No release plans	76	403	479
Not ascertained	2	6	8
Total	109	421	530

qualification for release, since likelihood of harm and degree of mental impairment correspond roughly to the two principal legal justifications for involuntary confinement: the police power of the state to protect itself against harm and *parens patriae*, the right of the state to assist those, who because of incapacity, may be unable to assist themselves. (A fuller discussion of this point is found in Ross [1959:130].) Those patients rated as likely to harm themselves or others if released will be considered as not qualified for release by reason of the police power. Those patients rated as severely mentally impaired will be considered to be not qualified for release by reason of *parens patriae*.

It may be objected that survey questions concerning degree of danger and mental impairment are overly simple and perhaps unreliable instruments for assessing the complex issues involved in estimating the patient's condition. It should be noted, however, that the psychiatrist or other official who answered the questions about the patient is the person *legally responsible* for the patient's welfare and is, therefore, in a position to give more than a casual evaluation. Although likelihood of danger and degree of mental impairment are admittedly only crude indices, these indices were administered in a uniform way (i.e., as questions on a standard questionnaire), they have face validity, and have never been demonstrated to be unreliable. In these respects, the indices compare favorably with the more traditional measure of the patient's condition: his psychiatric diagnosis. Psychiatric diagnoses are not made in a rigidly uniform manner, they do not have face validity, and they have been repeatedly demonstrated to be unreliable.[13] Under these conditions, the indices of danger and degree of mental impairment yield the best available estimate of the patient's qualifications for release.

The relationship between release plans and qualifications for release can be determined by noting the proportion of release plans within each impairment category, after excluding those cases which were rated as likely to harm themselves or others. Twenty cases from the receiving hospital sample and 129 cases from the transfer hospital sample were either rated as likely to harm themselves or others if released or not rated. (There were release plans for one patient in each of these two groups.) Table 6.3 shows the relationship between degree of mental impairment and release plans for the remainder of the sample: those patients rated as not likely to harm themselves or others.

This table shows that there is a very strong association between release plans and impairment in the receiving hospitals; the proportion of patients for whom there are release plans drops from 100% in the category "None or Minimal" to 7% in the category "Severe." In the transfer hospitals, the association is much weaker: Of those patients rated in the categories "None or Minimal, only 29% were reported with release plans. The proportion drops to 0% for those patients rated as severely impaired. The fact that the differences between release plans in the receiving and transfer hospitals does not disappear when patient quali-

---

[13]For a review, see Beck (1962).

TABLE 6.3.   Release Plans and Degree of Impairment of Patients Rated Not Likely to Harm Themselves or Others[a]

	Degree of impairment				
	None or minimal	Mild	Moderate	Severe	Total
Receiving hospitals					
Release plans	5(100%)	16(55%)	8(21%)	1(07%)	30
No release plans	0	13	30	14	57
Total	5	29	38	15	87

	Degree of impairment					
	None or minimal	Mild	Moderate	Severe	NA	Total
Transfer hospitals						
Release plans	5(29%)	4(7%)	2(2%)	0(0%)	0	11
No release plans	12	52	122	86	3	275
Total	17	56	124	86	3	286

[a]Omitted from this table are 148 patients rated as likely to harm self or others and 9 patients who were not rated as to release plans or likelihood of harm.

fications for release are introduced suggests that social contingencies (such as the patient's financial status, the availabililty of nursing homes, etc.) may be important in release.

Two contingencies that may be related to the differing rates of release plans are the age and length of confinement of the patients in each type of hospital as shown in Table 6.4. Fifty-five per cent of the patients in the transfer hospital sample were over 60 years of age, and only 10% of the patients in the receiving hospital were older than 60. Fifty-three per cent of the patients in the transfer hospitals have been confined for 10 years or longer, and only 18% of the patients in the receiving hospital have been confined for this long. It is conceivable that the ages and lengths of confinement of the patients, rather than differences in release policies, may account for the difference in the release plans rates.

One way of determining the effect of age and length of confinement on release is to determine if patients over 60 or those who have been confined for longer than 10 years are overrepresented in the group of "qualified" patients for whom there are no release plans. In the receiving hospital sample in Table 6.5, this is not the case: Patients over 60, or confined longer than 10 years, or both, represent only 5%, 9.5%, and 9.5%, respectively, of the group of qualified patients for whom there is no release plans ($N = 42$). These are roughly the same proportions as these age and confinement groups in the total receiving hospital sample.

TABLE 6.4.   Age and Length of Confinement of Patients in Receiving and Transfer Hospitals

Age	Length of confinement		Total
	Less than 10 years	10 years or more	
Receiving hospitals			
Under 60	85(78%)	13(12%)	98
60 or more	4(4%)	7(6%)	11
Total			109(100%)
Transfer hospitals			
Under 60	87(21%)	104(25%)	191
60 or more	111(26%)	119(28%)	230
Total			421(100%)

TABLE 6.5.   Age and Length of Confinement of Qualified Patients for Whom There Are No Release Plans

Age	Length of confinement			
	Receiving hospitals		Transfer hospitals	
	Less than 10 years	10 years or more	Less than 10 years	10 years or more
Under 60	32(76%)	4(10%)	43(23%)	85(46%)
60 or more	2(5%)	4(10%)	31(17%)	27(15%)
Total	42(100%)		186(100%)	

In the transfer hospital sample, however, patients confined more than 10 years are overrepresented in the group of qualified patients for whom there are no release plans. Patients over 60, or confined longer than 10 years, or both, constitute 17%, 46%, and 15%, respectively, of the qualified patients for whom there are no release plans but 25%, 26%, and 28% of the total transfer hospitals sample. Since the proportion of patients under 60 years of age but confined longer than 10 years is almost twice as great among the qualified patients for whom there are no release plans than it is in the sample as a whole, length of confinement is suggested as an important contingency for release in the transfer hospitals.

If a shorter length of confinement (2 years) is taken as a cutting point, the effect of length of confinement on release plans can be seen even in the treatment and release-oriented receiving hospitals. In Table 6.6, the relationship between release plans and impairment for short- and long-term patients in the receiving

TABLE 6.6. Release Plans, Degree of Mental Impairment, and Length of Hospitalization for Patients in Receiving Hospitals Sample Who Were Rated as Unlikely to Harm Themselves or Others

	Degree of mental impairment		
	None, minimal, or mild	Moderate or severe	Total
Length of hospitalization: 0–2 years			
Release plans	15(72%)	6(16%)	21
No release plans	6	32	38
Total	21	38	59
Length of hospitalization: 2 or more years			
Release plans	6(46%)	3(20%)	9
No release plans	7	12	19
Totals	13	15	28

hospitals is shown. (As in Table 6.6, the 20 patients rated as likely to harm themselves or others are excluded as are two patients for whom length of confinement was not ascertained.) According to Table 6.6, for those patients (rated as unlikely to harm themselves or others) who have been in the receiving hospitals for less than 2 years, there are release plans for 72% of the slightly impaired and 16% of the moderately and severely impaired. For those patients who had been in the receiving hospitals for more than 2 years, there are release plans for only 46% of the slightly impaired and for 20% of the moderately and severely impaired. The proportion of patients for whom there were release plans is very low for patients rated as moderately or severely impaired in both short- and long-term groups. For the slightly impaired, however, the proportion of patients for whom there were release plans drops from 72% of the short-term patients to 46% of the long-term patients, suggesting that release chances decrease for long-term patients whatever their qualifications for release. This finding provides support for the idea current among mental health workers that long confinement can, in itself, reduce patients' chances for discharge.

This section has presented data to test the hypothesis that social, rather than psychiatric, contingencies may be crucial in release plans for mental patients. Ratings of the likelihood that patients would harm themselves or others if released and ratings of the degree of mental impairment were employed as indices of psychiatric contingencies. The social contingencies were type of hospital, age, and length of continuous confinement.

The findings strongly support the initial hypothesis. The treatment and release-oriented receiving hospital were found to have a much greater proportion of release plans than the custody-oriented transfer hospitals. This difference does

not disappear when differences in the qualifications of the patients are introduced. The majority of patients who appear qualified for release from a
medical and legal point of view, but for whom there are no release plans, are
patients whose age or length of confinement appear to be significant contingencies. Since age and long confinement would tend to make patients dependent on
their families and community, the importance of these variables suggest that the
community's acceptance of its former members may be a crucial contingency in
release.[14]

The data presented here indicate that there is a large proportion of the patient
population, 43%, whose presence in the hospital cannot readily be explained in
terms of their psychiatric condition. Their presence suggests the putative character of the societal reaction to deviance, and that for at least a near-majority of
the patients, their status is largely ascribed rather than achieved. All of the
findings taken together point to the usefulness of an analysis of career contingencies in the social mobility of mental patients, quite distinct from considerations of the dynamics of "mental illness."

---

[14]The effect of the community's attitude is increased in those hospitals that maintain an informal
policy of retaining marginal patients unless someone in the community is willing to take the
responsibility for them. The existence of such policies was noted in Gainford's (1956) comments
(1956) on *Report on Texas Hospitals and Institutions*: "In Texas, as in other states, it was a rule in
state hospitals that no patient could be released unless he had a place to go to.'''

Users and Nonusers of a Student Psychiatric Clinic[1]

7

INTRODUCTION

CHAPTER 6 reports two studies of the societal reaction to residual rule-breaking. This chapter reports a study not of the societal reaction but of personal reactions. How do individuals react to their own ''psychiatric symptoms''? The findings suggest that there is a difference in readiness to define themselves in need of psychiatric assistance among different groups, and that this readiness, somewhat more than the number of symptoms, leads people into psychiatric treatment. This study could be interpreted as dealing with the process of self-labeling.

Sociological studies have repeatedly shown that voluntary use of psychiatric clinics is highly correlated with social variables such as education, income, and occupational level.[2] Since nonusers are not included in the research design of these studies, however, there remains some ambiguity in the interpretation of these findings. Two opposing interpretations are possible, in fact. The first is that a social stratum is overrepresented in a clinic because there is more psychiatric illness in that stratum. The second is that there is approximately the same amount of illness in all the strata, but that there is a differential reaction to illness, resulting in overrepresentation in some strata and underrepresentation in others.

[1]This study was supported by grants from the Graduate Research Committees of the University of Wisconsin and the University of California, Santa Barbara. The assistance of the psychiatrists in the Student Health Service of the University of Wisconsin and their director, Dr. Herman Gladstone, is gratefully acknowledged as is the assistance of Arnold Silverman, University of Wisconsin.

[2]Gurin, Veroff, and Feld (1960:334–338), Schaffer and Myers (1954); Imber *et al.* (1955); Winder and Hesko (1956); Sullivan *et al.* (1958); Moses and Shana (1961).

This ambiguity runs like a thread through most studies of social medicine and also in the study of deviant behavior (e.g., in the interpretation of social differentials in crime rates) and represents, therefore, a fundamental problem in the sociology of medicine and of deviant behavior.

The purpose of the present research is to clarify this problem by including both users and nonusers in a study of the utilization of a student psychiatric clinic in a large university. A survey was made of users and nonusers on a standard, self-administered questionnaire, which included items concerning the student's social characteristics, university activities, and a checklist of the types of problems that students typically presented at the psychiatric clinic. As a crude index of the degree of psychiatric stress, the total number of problems that the student checked was used. Before examining the relationships among psychiatric stress, social characteristics, and use of the clinic, some of the details concerning the survey are considered.

TECHNIQUE

To determine whether the clientele of the University of Wisconsin Psychiatric Infirmary had any special characteristics, two surveys were conducted. The first included all student applicants to the clinic during the spring semester, 1962. Of 88 applicants, three students did not return the questionnaire, and two refused to complete it, giving a completion rate of 94%.[3] The second surveyed the population from which the clinic applicants came, the University of Wisconsin student body. A 2% systematic sample drawn from the student directory yielded 400 names. A questionnaire mailed to these students was returned by 309, giving a response rate for the nonclinic group of 77%.[4]

The items on the questionnaires administered to the two groups were almost identical. In the clinic group, the questionnaire was called Problems of Students Using the Psychiatric Infirmary. In the nonclinic group, the intent of the questionnaire was disguised (the title used was Inventory of Student Problems). By checking age, birthplace, and other characteristics it was ascertained that no student was included in both samples.

The frequency distributions of the clinic and nonclinic samples will now be examined for differences in social background, social position, and number of presenting problems. (Summary measures of the association between these variables and clinic use are presented in Table 7.9, column "a".) The age and sex distributions of the samples of clinic applicants and the student body differ only

[3]During the semester, there were actually 114 applicants to the clinic, but a sequence of 26 were inadvertantly not given the questionnaire. Since there was no obvious bias in this omission, it should not affect the typicality of the sample.

[4]Sex, school class, and region of home address of the nonreturners were ascertained from the directory and compared with these characteristics of the returners. The nonreturners, with one slight exception, did not appear to differ significantly from the returners. The exception was foreign students: These comprised 6% of the nonreturners and only 1% of the returners.

slightly. Older students are somewhat overrepresented in the clinic sample (52% in the clinic and 48% in the student body were over 21), and females are somewhat overrepresented (41% in the clinic, 35% in the student body). The relationship between clinic use and the education and occupation of the applicants' fathers is somewhat stronger. Applicants whose fathers received at least some college education are overrepresented (63% in the clinic, 52% in the student body) as well as those whose fathers held high prestige occupations (over .65 on the Hatt-Reiss scale of occupational prestige: 57% in the clinic, 46% in the student body). Clinic use is also related to the size of the city and the region of the United States in which the applicants attended high school. Students who attended high school in a city of 100,000 or more constitute 40% of the clinic sample but only 22% of the student body sample. Region of birthplace is also related. Students attending high school in the Northeast region of the United States constitute 31% of the clinic sample but only 13% of the student body sample.

Turning from background characteristics to current activities, college major, extracurricular activities, number of close friends, and religious participation are discussed. Students in the social and behavioral sciences and humanities are overrepresented in the clinic (51% in the clinic as against 30% of the student body), and students in the natural sciences and professional schools are underrepresented (37% of the clinic sample and 58% of the student body sample). In regard to number of close friends in Madison, the clinic and student body distributions differ only slightly except for those having five or more friends. In this category, the clinic group is underrepresented. The relationship between clinic use and extracurricular activities is more linear: Students listing no extracurricular activities are overrepresented in the clinic sample, students with one or two activities are proportionately represented, and students with three or more activities are underrepresented.

Of all the variables considered, the strongest relationship is with religion and religious participation. Representation in the clinic sample varies directly with degree of religious participation: Students who never participate are greatly overrepresented in the clinic sample, with 38% responding in this way but only 9% of the students in the student body sample never participating. The degree of overrepresentation decreases with increasing religious participation, with students who participate regularly (weekly or more) greatly underrepresented in the clinic (20% as compared with 46% in the student body).

The church to which the student is affiliated is also related to clinic use. Protestants and Catholics are underrepresented in the clinic relative to their numbers in the student body, and Jews, nonaffiliated, and other (Greek Orthodox, Moslem, and Buddhist), are overrepresented. The nonaffiliated are the group most strongly overrepresented: 37% of the clinic sample as against 13% of the student body sample, almost three times the rate in the clinic as in the student body.

By examining the characteristics of the applicants to the clinic and the student body of which they are part, we have sought to isolate the characteristics of persons who comprise a sizeable proportion of the applicants to the clinic but only a small part of the student body. Obviously overrepresented are persons with the following backgrounds: their fathers are educated, and have high prestige occupations, they themselves are Jewish, nonaffiliated, or belong to a minority religion. Their place of birth is large and located in the Northeastern part of the United States. In terms of their current activities, members of this group major in the humanities, social, or behavioral science, engage in few extracurricular activities, have somewhat fewer close friends than other students, and participate slightly or not at all in religious activities.

The next question is to determine the extent to which this group is overrepresented in treatment because its members have more psychiatric illness, by introducing the number of personal problems as a test variable. If, after controlling for the number of personal problems, the relationship between the social characteristics of the students and the use of the clinic disappears, then we can reason that the original relationship has been explained by the problems of the applicants; the members of certain strata are overrepresented in the clinic because they have more problems than other groups in the student body. If the relationships do not disappear, which is the case, then we must seek other interpretations of the original relationships.

The items in the problems checklist were suggested by the infirmary psychiatrists as being the kinds of problems students typically presented during the first interview. A total of 58 problems were included and were listed under the headings: Studies, Social Life, Money and Work, Emotional Problems, Physical Illness and Other Problems, Family, and Religion and Morality. The first item under each of these headings is given below as examples of the types of problems included.

Studies	22.	Read but it doesn't sink in.
Social Life	38.	Can't get along with my roommate.
Money and Work	49.	Part-time work interferes with my studies.
Emotional Problems	53.	Panicked in an examination and had to leave the room.
Physical Illness	66.	Chronic indigestion, heartburn.
Family	75.	Worry about divorce of parents.
Religion and Morality	82.	Confusion over beliefs learned at home and those of people here.

Table 7.1 shows the distribution of problems in the clinic and student body samples. The number of problems is strongly related to use of the clinic; about 59% of the clinic sample have 10 or more problems, but only 35% of the student body sample have this many problems. This is a larger association than was shown by any of the social characteristics taken singly, with the exception of religious participation and religion. It is possible, therefore, that the members of

TABLE 7.1   Number of Problems in Student Body and Clinic Samples

	Clinic		Student body	
Number of Problems	%	N	%	N
0	2	(2)	8	(25)
1–3	13	(11)	24	(73)
4–6	12	(10)	17	(53)
7–9	12	(10)	16	(50)
10–12	25	(21)	14	(43)
13–19	27	(22)	15	(46)
20–26	6	(5)	5	(14)
27 or more	0	(0)	1	(4)
NA	2	(2)	0	(0)
Total number		(83)		(308)

the overrepresented strata use the clinic because they have more problems than other students. If this were the case, the original relationship between social characteristics and clinic use would disappear or be reduced when the number of problems is controlled.

In the following tables, control for the number of problems is introduced by dividing the clinic and student body samples into those with fewer than 10 problems and those with 10 problems or more. Of the social background variables, we consider father's education and occupational prestige and the region and population of the city where the student attended high school. Table 7.2 shows the distribution of father's level of education for the clinic and student body samples among those with few and many problems.

The association between father's education and clinic use exists within both low problem and high problem groups. The strength of the association, however, is greater in the few problems group and smaller in the many problems group. This pattern is repeated in all of the remaining social background tables (tables 7.3, 7.4, and 7.5).

For the current activities variables, since the same pattern is repeated, tables will be presented for only the three strongest relationships, School Major, Religious Participation, and Religion (see Tables 7.6, 7.7, and 7.8). The recurring pattern in these tables appears to be first, the original relationship does not disappear when number of problems is introduced as a test variable, and second, in most of the tables, the association changes in the partial tables by becoming stronger in the few problems group and weaker in the many problems group.

Table 7.9 presents summary measures of association between students' characteristics and clinic use. If we ignore the three variables that are only weakly associated with clinic use (age, sex, and number of close friends), the pattern of a stronger association in the few problems group occurs with every variable except religion.

TABLE 7.2   Father's Education in Clinic and Student Body Samples[a]

| Education | Few problems (0–9) | | | | Many problems (10 or more) | | | |
| | Clinic | | Student body | | Clinic | | Student body | |
	%	N	%	N	%	N	%	N
Less than high school	27	(9)	26	(53)	17	(8)	18	(19)
High school	3	(1)	24	(48)	21	(10)	23	(24)
Some college	42	(14)	36	(73)	35	(17)	42	(44)
Completed graduate school	24	(8)	11	(23)	25	(12)	15	(16)
NA	3	(1)	2	(4)	2	(1)	3	(3)
Total number		(33)		(201)		(48)		(106)

[a]Two students in the clinic sample and one in the student body sample did not check the problems section and are excluded in this table and the subsequent tables.

TABLE 7.3   Father's Occupation in Clinic and Student Body Samples

| Occupation | Few problems (0–9) | | | | Many problems (10 or more) | | | |
| | Clinic | | Student body | | Clinic | | Student body | |
	%	N	%	N	%	N	%	N
Low	9	(3)	30	(61)	19	(9)	13	(14)
Medium	18	(6)	14	(29)	13	(6)	25	(27)
High	70	(23)	51	(102)	60	(29)	58	(61)
NA	3	(1)	5	(9)	8	(4)	4	(4)
Total number		(33)		(201)		(48)		(106)

TABLE 7.4   Population of City in Which Student Attended High School in Clinic and Student Body Samples

| Population | Few problems (0–9) | | | | Many problems (10 or more) | | | |
| | Clinic | | Student body | | Clinic | | Student body | |
	%	N	%	N	%	N	%	N
Fewer than 10,000	3	(1)	28	(56)	8	(4)	18	(19)
Fewer than 100,000	24	(8)	31	(62)	35	(17)	39	(41)
100,000 or more	63	(21)	37	(75)	42	(20)	35	(38)
NA	9	(3)	4	(8)	15	(7)	8	(8)
Total number		(33)		(201)		(48)		(106)

TABLE 7.5 Birthplace: Region in Clinic and Student Body Samples

Birthplace	Few problems (0–9)				Many problems (10 or more)			
	Clinic		Student body		Clinic		Student body	
	%	N	%	N	%	N	%	N
Northeast U.S.	55	(11)	13	(26)	21	(10)	10	(11)
Southwest U.S.	12	(4)	6	(13)	10	(5)	6	(6)
Northcentral U.S.	52	(17)	77	(154)	60	(29)	78	(83)
Non-U.S.	3	(1)	3	(7)	4	(2)	6	(6)
NA		(0)	0	(1)	4	(2)		(0)
Total number		(33)		(201)		(48)		(106)

TABLE 7.6 School Major in Clinic and Student Body Samples

School major	Few problems (0–9)				Many problems (10 or more)			
	Clinic		Student body		Clinic		Student body	
	%	N	%	N	%	N	%	N
Humanities	21	(7)	13	(26)	35	(17)	18	(19)
Social and behavioral science	39	(13)	15	(31)	10	(5)	16	(17)
Professional schools and other	27	(9)	49	(98)	44	(21)	46	(49)
Natural sciences	3	(1)	16	(33)	8	(4)	10	(11)
NA	9	(3)	7	(13)	2	(1)	9	(10)
Total number		(33)		(201)		(48)		(106)

TABLE 7.7 Religious Participation in Clinic and Student Body Samples

Religious participation	Few problems (0–9)				Many problems (10 or more)			
	Clinic		Student body		Clinic		Student body	
	%	N	%	N	%	N	%	N
Never	33	(11)	8	(17)	49	(21)	9	(10)
1–4 / year	27	(9)	17	(34)	23	(11)	25	(27)
5–24 / year	21	(7)	24	(48)	12	(6)	26	(28)
Weekly or more	15	(5)	50	(101)	21	(10)	37	(39)
NA	3	(33)	0	(1)		(0)	1	(2)
Total number				(201)		(48)		(106)

TABLE 7.8   Religion in Clinic and Student Body Samples

| | Few problems (0–9) | | | | Many problems (10 or more) | | | |
| | Clinic | | Student body | | Clinic | | Student body | |
Religion	%	N	%	N	%	N	%	N
Protestant	27	(9)	53	(106)	29	(14)	58	(61)
Catholic	12	(4)	23	(47)	8	(4)	17	(18)
Jewish	24	(8)	10	(19)	14	(7)	10	(15)
Nonaffiliated	27	(9)	12	(25)	46	(22)	14	(11)
Other	3	(1)		(0)	2	(1)		(0)
NA	6	(2)	2	(4)		(0)	1	(1)
Total number		(33)		(201)		(48)		(106)

Two questions need to be raised about the findings at this point. First, to what extent are the results influenced by the method of collecting data? Since the university clinic is not the only source of psychiatric services for students, it could be argued that the local students tend to go to psychiatrists not connected with the university. Conversely, students from outside of Madison or outside the state would be more likely to use the university clinic than to go to local psychiatrists. To check this possibility, the responses of the students in the nonclinic sample to this question were scanned: "Have you gotten help for any of these problems?" (the problems which they had checked). Removing the few cases in which the student signified that he had gone to a psychiatrist (1% of the sample) only slightly attenuates the correlations just reported, suggesting that the findings are not an artifact of the method of gathering data.

The second question concerns the interrelations between the independent variables found to be correlated with clinic use. Are these variables highly intercorrelated so that all the different variables are simply different aspects of the same underlying pattern, or does each variable independently account for some of the variance? To answer this question, the method of "path analysis" was used. It was found that the coefficient of multiple correlation for all of the 10 independent variables was C. = .42, and that the bulk of this relationship could be expressed by only three of the variables: Religion, C. = .18, religious participation, C. = .13, and number of problems, C. = .11. The correlations between clinic use and the other variables, therefore, can be considered to be represented by these three variables.

DISCUSSION

The findings show that there are persons with certain social backgrounds and current social positions who are overrepresented among clinic applicants relative to their representation in the student body. Since we found that use of the clinic was strongly associated with number of personal problems, we sought to explain

TABLE 7.9 Association of Students' Characteristics with Use of Psychiatric Clinic[a]

Characteristic	Group	(a) Total association	(b) Partial association (few problems group)	(c) Partial association (many problems group)
Age	21 and over	.05	.12	.13
Sex	Female	.12	− .25	.21
Father's education	Beyond high school	.25	.40	.20
Father's occupation	High prestige	.25	.30	.20
Birthplace: City size	100,000 or more	.34	.57	.19
Birthplace: Region	Northeast and Southeast	.46	.55	.49
School major	Humanities and social science	.38	.64	.26
Number of close friends	Four or less	.24	.21	.24
Number of extracurricular activities	None	.32	.34	.29
Religious participation	Four times a year or less	.63	.66	.57
Religion	Jewish, nonaffiliated or "other"	.66	.64	.67
Number of personal problems	10 or more	.47		

[a]The coefficient of association is Yule's Q, computed from fourfold tables in which the students' characteristics have been reduced to dichotomies. A positive coefficient indicates that the group named under the heading "Group" is overrepresented in the clinic.

122

the use of the clinic by these persons by the fact that they have more personal problems than other students. When the number of personal problems is controlled, however, the original relationships between social characteristics do not disappear. We, therefore, must attempt to explain the original relationship in some other manner.

To pose the problem differently: Since the findings indicate that the over-representation of certain social strata cannot be explained by pointing to more illness in those strata, is there some *social* process which could lead to the high correlation between social characteristics and clinic use? In the following interpretation, our findings concerning clinic utilization are explained in terms of elementary collective behavior, by considering some of the clinic users to be part of a psychiatric public, and the use of the clinic by the remainder to be the convergence of individual lines of action, which may be called "mass behavior."

Students of collective behavior usually treat mass behavior as the extreme individualistic pole of a continuum with social movements at the other extreme.[5] Between these two extremes fall crowds, which are more organized than the mass, and publics, which are still more organized. Mass behavior is not part of a social process; it has been defined as the convergence of a large number of independent actions made on the basis of individual impulses and feelings. This definition appears applicable to some persons seeking medical services; through a process of trial and error, and apparently accidental events, they end up as applicants for a medical service.

It has recently been pointed out, however, that the selection of medical services is not accidental or random for some patients but depends on the actions of organized communities or other social groups. In his discussion of the "lay referral system," Freidson (1960) notes that the individual's choice of physicians may be mediated by members of the community to which he belongs. Writing specifically about the practice of psychotherapy, Kadushin (1962) argues that special coteries, "the friends and supporters of psychotherapy and psychoanalysis," not only serve as channels of recruitment but also function as a part of the treatment itself, serving to bridge the social distance between the client and the professional. To the extent that membership in such coteries is stable, this type of group may be appropriately classified as a "psychiatric following," which is a type of incipient social movement (Turner and Killian, 1957:454–457).

Both the "lay referral system" and the "friends and supporters of psychotherapy and psychoanalysis" would appear to be made up of persons in direct or mediated contact, who influence one another by word-of-mouth information, suggestions, and evaluations. In addition to such direct contact groups, however, there appears to be a much larger group (which includes these coteries and many

[5]Cf. Turner and Killian (1957).

other persons in addition) that is involved in the process of seeking medical assistance.

Although the conception of a *public* is defined somewhat differently in the standard literature, it is defined for the present purposes as "a dispersed group of individuals who are located in the same channels of communication, who therefore develop consensus over an issue, and whose actions with respect to the issue impinge on a focal point in the social structure."[6] The members of the group that is overrepresented in the psychiatric clinic are persons of similar social background and current social activities and who are probably involved, therefore, in the same kinds of social milieux. Having college-trained parents, not involved in religious activities, of Eastern, urban, professional backgrounds, they share similar social, cultural, and political activities. Of particular significance, they probably are exposed to the same kinds of educational and mass media influences: sophisticated fiction and political commentary and "serious" forms of entertainment, news, and special features in the mass media.

It could be argued, therefore, that members of this public are the persons most affected by the mental health movement. Prior studies of the impact of mass media mental health campaigns seem to indicate that only a small segment of the population accepts the major premises of the mental health ideology.[7] *The psychiatric public, therefore, is that segment of the population that takes for granted the reality and, secondarily, the respectability of mental illness*. Since the majority in the larger society do not take this issue for granted, this perspective is in need of constant support. In the psychiatric public, the reality of mental illness is continuously reaffirmed in those portions of the mass media to which this public is exposed and in ordinary social interaction among its members. But this is to say that a medical definition of personal problems is more likely to be sustained among members of the psychiatric public.

By the same token, the majority of Americans are not psychiatrically sophisticated. For them, personal problems are not defined as psychiatric until they are overwhelming. Even then, resorting to psychiatric services is avoided as long as possible. These persons would tend to reach the clinic, therefore, only in a crisis, which can be considered mass behavior. The data shown in Tables 7.2–7.9 provide support for this interpretation. Members of the psychiatric mass (i.e., persons of Midwestern, rural, Protestant background, etc.) tend to be greatly

[6]Current definitions of the concept of a *public*, which stress debate over an issue, seem unnecessarily restrictive and more suitable for the discussion of one special type of public, the political public. For the definition used here, the author has drawn upon the broader concept of *public* suggested by John Dewey (1927:15–19). Mills used the concept similarly: "Political publics may be located by the publications they read and the organizations they support [1948: p. 14]."

[7]The Cummings (1957:86–87), for example, found that an intensive mental health educational campaign had virtually no effect in low education groups but appeared to cause shifts in opinions and attitudes among persons with at least a high school education. Education and income are also correlated with "readiness for self-referral [Gurin, Veroff, and Feld, 1960:278]." For data showing the association of information and attitude toward mental illness and psychiatrists with income and education, see Nunally (1961).

underrepresented in the clinic among persons with few problems. Among persons with many problems, however, the proportions of these persons in the clinic tend to approximate their proportions in the student body.

Having suggested that the clinic clientele can be divided into members of the mass and members of the psychiatric public, we may now consider one implication of this finding. Assuming that elementary collective behavior does play a part in bringing persons to the clinic, how great a part of the clinic clientele can be attributed to it? Suppose as a crude index of membership in the psychiatric public, we take low religious participation. As the excess of clinic applicants contributed by collective behavior in the psychiatric public, we take those applicants with few (0–9) problems and low (less than four times a year) religious participation. Even if we consider this entire group to arise out of the psychiatric public, it constitutes, according to Table 7.7, only 24% of the clinic sample, a rather small proportion of the whole.

It should be remembered, however, that this study has concerned only *applicants* to the clinic and not persons under treatment. Since at this clinic persons actually in treatment make up the great bulk of the clinic work load, it is important to consider the possible effects of the mass–public differential on staying in treatment in addition to application to the clinic. As in other clinics, there is considerable drop-out, perhaps as high as two-thirds of the applicants, after the first several interviews. Prior studies have established that it is the more sophisticated persons from highly educated, high income groups who stay in treatment.[8] It does not seem unreasonable to argue, therefore, that it is the members of the psychiatric public who continue in treatment and the members of the mass who drop out. If this is the case, members of the psychiatric public, who probably constitute less than a quarter of the applicants, may well make up the majority of persons in treatment. Stating the argument in a different way, we are suggesting that the presence of the bulk of the clinic's clientele may be explained less by disease processes than by elementary collective behavior.

Since this study was only exploratory, the explanation of clinic use in terms of collective behavior cannot be said to have been demonstrated, but only suggested for purposes of further research and discussion. To validate the analysis suggested here, future studies would need more refined measures of psychiatric stress, such as measures of the type and intensity of personal problems as well as indices of membership in an organized public: referral path, exposure to psychiatric content in the mass media, and attribution of consensus on psychiatric matters to members of one's social circle.

CONCLUSION

In this study of characteristics of users and nonusers of a psychiatric clinic, it was found that the overrepresentation of certain social strata in the use of the clinic is not explained by the presence of more "illness" in these strata. The

---

[8]See the second, third, and fourth studies listed in Footnote 2.

correlation between social characteristics and clinic use is weaker, however, among persons having a larger number of personal problems and stronger among those with few problems. These findings are interpreted to mean that persons who come to the clinic with few problems tend to be members of a psychiatric public, whose exposure to the mass media and other members of the psychiatric public lead them to define these problems psychiatrically. This exposure also causes and sustains the motivation and information about psychiatric services, which leads them to take these problems to the clinic. It is suggested that this interpretation should be tested by introducing measures of membership in a psychiatric public and more refined measures of psychiatric stress.

Negotiating Reality: Notes on Power in the Assessment of Responsibility[1]

8

INTRODUCTION

THIS chapter shows the application of labeling ideas to two particular contexts: the offices of a defense lawyer and of a practicing psychiatrist. Labeling concepts are very abstract. In order to understand their implications, it is necessary to observe their effects in concrete, particular events. The labeling that the psychiatrist is doing in the interview below is very subtle; it is not completely articulated in words and is probably outside the awareness of both the patient and the psychiatrist. Yet, its effects are very constraining. The normalization being practiced by the defense lawyer is also mostly nonverbal. In his case, however, he is probably aware of what he is doing. This chapter provides a very detailed and explicit contrast between the processes of labeling and normalization.

The use of interrogation to reconstruct parts of an individual's past history is a common occurrence in human affairs. Reporters, jealous lovers, and policemen on the beat are often faced with the task of determining events in another person's life and the extent to which he was responsible for those events. The most dramatic use of interrogation to determine responsibility is in criminal trials. As in everyday life, criminal trials are concerned with both act and intent. Courts, in most cases,

[1]The author wishes to acknowledge the help of the following persons who criticized earlier drafts: Aaron Cicourel, Donald Cressey, Joan Emerson, Erving Goffman, Michael Katz, Lewis Kurke, Robert Levy, Sohan Lal Sharma, and Paul Weubben. The chapter was written during a fellowship provided by the Social Science Research Institute, University of Hawaii.

first determine whether the defendant performed a legally forbidden act. If it is found that he did so, the court then must decide whether he was "responsible" for the act. Reconstructive work of this type goes on less dramatically in a wide variety of other settings, as well. The social worker determining a client's eligibility for unemployment compensation, for example, seeks not only to establish that the client actually is unemployed, but that he has actively sought employment (i.e., that he himself is not responsible for being out of work).

This chapter contrasts two perspectives on the process of reconstructing past events for the purpose of fixing responsibility. The first perspective stems from the common sense notion that interrogation, when it is sufficiently skillful, is essentially neutral. Responsibility for past actions can be fixed absolutely and independently of the method of reconstruction. This perspective is held by the typical member of society, engaged in his day-to-day tasks. It is also held, in varying degrees, by most professional interrogators. The basic working doctrine is one of *absolute* responsibility. This point of view actually entails the comparison of two different kinds of items: first, the fixing of actions and intentions, and second, comparing these actions and intentions to some predetermined criteria of responsibility. The basic premise of the doctrine of absolute responsibility is that both actions and intentions, on the one hand, and the criteria of responsibility, on the other, are absolute in that they can be assessed independently of social context.[2]

An alternative approach follows from the sociology of knowledge. From this point of view, the reality within which members of society conduct their lives is largely of their own construction.[3] Since much of reality is a construction, there may be multiple realities, existing side by side, in harmony or in competition. It follows, if one maintains this stance, that the assessment of responsibility involves the construction of reality by members: construction both of actions and intentions, on the one hand, and of criteria of responsibility, on the other. The former process, the continuous reconstruction of the normative order, has long been the focus of sociological concern.[4] The discussion in this chapter is limited, for the most part, to the former process, the way in which actions and intentions are constructed in the act of assessing responsibility.

My purpose is to argue that responsibility is at least partly a product of social structure. The alternative to the doctrine of absolute responsibility is that of relative responsibility: The assessment of responsibility always includes a process of negotiation. In this process, responsibility is in part constructed by the negotiating parties. To illustrate this thesis, excerpts from two dialogues of negotiation will be discussed: a real psychotherapeutic interview and an interview between a

---

[2]The doctrine of absolute responsibility is clearly illustrated in psychiatric and legal discussions of the issue of "criminal responsibility" (i.e., the use of mental illness as an excuse from criminal conviction). An example of the assumption of absolute criteria of responsibility is found in the following quotation: "The finding that someone is criminally responsible means to the psychiatrist that the criminal must change his behavior before he can resume his position in society. *This injunction is dictated not by morality, but, so to speak, by reality* [Sachar, 1963:emphasis added]."

[3]Cf. Berger and Luckmann (1966).

[4]The classic treatment of this issue is found in Durkheim (1915).

defense attorney and his client, taken from a work of fiction. Before presenting these excerpts, it is useful to review some prior discussions of negotiation, the first in courts of law, the second in medical diagnosis.[5]

The negotiation of pleas in criminal courts, sometimes referred to as "bargain justice," has been frequently noted by observers of legal processes.[6] The defense attorney or (in many cases, apparently) the defendant himself strikes a bargain with the prosecutor—a plea of guilty will be made provided that the prosecutor will reduce the charge. For example, a defendant arrested on suspicion of armed robbery may arrange to plead guilty to the charge of unarmed robbery. The prosecutor obtains ease of conviction from the bargain, the defendant, leniency.

Although no explicit estimates are given, it appears from observers' reports that the great majority of criminal convictions are negotiated. Newman (1966) states:

> A major characteristic of criminal justice administration, particularly in jurisdictions charac-
> terized by legislatively fixed sentences, is charge reduction to elicit pleas of guilty. Not only does
> the efficient functioning of criminal justice rest upon a high proportion of guilty pleas, but plea
> bargaining is closely linked with attempts to individualize justice, to obtain certain desirable
> conviction consequences, and to avoid undesirable ones such as "undeserved" mandatory
> sentences [p. 76].

It would appear that the bargaining process is accepted as routine. In the three jurisdictions Newman studied, there were certain meeting places where the defendant, his client, and a representative of the prosecutor's office routinely met to negotiate the plea. It seems clear that in virtually all but the most unusual cases, the interested parties expected to, and actually did, negotiate the plea.

From these comments on the routine acceptance of plea bargaining in the courts, one may expect that this process would be relatively open and unambiguous. Apparently, however, there is some tension between the fact of bargaining and moral expectations concerning justice. Newman refers to this tension by citing two contradictory statements: an actual judicial opinion, "Justice and liberty are not the subjects of bargaining and barter"; and an off-the-cuff statement by another judge. "All law is compromise," A clear example of this tension is provided by an excerpt from a trial and Newman's comments on it.

> The following questions were asked of a defendant after he had pleaded guilty to unarmed
> robbery when the original charge was armed robbery. This reduction is common, and the judge
> was fully aware that the plea was negotiated:
>
> | Judge: | You want to plead guilty to robbery unarmed? |
> | Defendant: | Yes, Sir. |
> | Judge: | Your plea of guilty is free and voluntary? |
> | Defendant: | Yes, Sir. |
> | Judge: | No one has promised you anything? |
> | Defendant: | No. |

---

[5]A sociological application of the concept of *negotiation*, in a different context, is found in Strauss *et al.* (1963:147–169).

[6]Newman (1966) reports a study in this area, together with a review of earlier work, in "The Negotiated Plea" Part 3 of the complete work.

Judge:	No one has induced you to plead guilty?
Defendant:	No.
Judge:	You're pleading guilty because you are guilty?
Defendant:	Yes.
Judge:	I'll accept your plea of guilty to robbery unarmed and refer it to the probation department for a report and for sentencing Dec. 28 [p. 83].

The delicacy of the relationship between appearance and reality is apparently confusing, even for the sociologist–observer. Newman's comment on this exchange has an Alice-in-Wonderland quality: "This is a routine procedure designed to satisfy the statutory requirement and is not intended to disguise the process of charge reduction [p. 83]." If we put the tensions between the different realities aside for the moment, we can say that there is an explicit process of negotiation between the defendant and the prosecution that is a part of the legal determination of guilt or innocence, or in the terms used here, the assessment of responsibility.

In medical diagnosis, a similar process of negotiation occurs but is much less self-conscious than plea bargaining. The English psychoanalyst, Michael Balint, refers to this process as one of "offers and responses":

> Some of the people who, for some reason or other, find it difficult to cope with problems of their lives resort to becoming ill. If the doctor has the opportunity of seeing them in the first phases of their being ill, i.e. before they settle down to a definite "organized" illness, he may observe that the patients, so to speak, offer or propose various illnesses, and that they have to go on offering new illnesses until between doctor and patient an agreement can be reached resulting in the acceptance by both of them of one of the illnesses as justified [1957:18].

Balint gives numerous examples indicating that patients propose reasons for their coming to the doctor that are rejected, one by one, by the physician, who makes counterproposals until an "illness" acceptable to both parties is found. If "definition of the situation" is substituted for "illness," Balint's observations become relevant to a wide variety of transactions, including the kind of interrogation just discussed. The fixing of responsibility is a process in which the client offers definitions of the situation to which the interrogator responds. After a series of offers and responses, a definition of the situation acceptable to both the client and the interrogator is reached.

Balint has observed that the negotiation process leads physicians to influence the outcome of medical examinations independently of the patient's condition. He refers to this process as the "apostolic function" of the doctor, arguing that the physician induces patients to have the kind of illness that the physician thinks is proper:

> Apostolic mission or function means in the first place that every doctor has a vague, but almost unshakably firm, idea of how a patient ought to behave when ill. Although this idea is anything but explicit and concrete, it is immensely powerful, and influences, as we have found, practically

---

[7]A description of the negotiations between patients in a tuberculosis sanitarium and their physicians is found in Roth (1963:48–59). Obviously, some cases are more susceptible to negotiation than others. Balint implies that the great majority of cases in medical practice are negotiated.

every detail of the doctor's work with his patients. It was almost as if every doctor had revealed knowledge of what was right and what was wrong for patients to expect and to endure, and further, as if he had a sacred duty to convert to his faith all the ignorant and unbelieving among his patients [216].

Implicit in this statement is the notion that interrogator and client have unequal power in determining the resultant definition of the situation. The interrogator's definition of the situation plays an important part in the joint definition of the situation which is finally negotiated. Moreover, his definition is more important than the client's in determining the final outcome of the negotiation, principally because he is well trained, secure, and self-confident in his role in the transaction, whereas the client is untutored, anxious, and uncertain about his role. Stated simply, the subject, because of these conditions, is likely to be susceptible to the influence of the interrogator.

Note that plea bargaining and the process of "offers and responses" in diagnosis differ in the degree of self-consciousness of the participants. In plea bargaining, the process is at least partly visible to the participants themselves. There appears to be some ambiguity about the extent to which the negotiation is morally acceptable to some of the commentators, but the parties to the negotiations appear to be aware that bargaining is going on and accept the process as such. The bargaining process in diagnosis, however, is much more subterranean. Certainly, neither physicians nor patients recognize the offers and responses process as being bargaining. There is no commonly accepted vocabulary for describing diagnostic bargaining, such as there is in the legal analogy (e.g., "copping out" or "copping a plea"). It may be that in legal processes there is some appreciation of the different kinds of reality (i.e., the difference between the public [official, legal] reality and private reality), whereas in medicine, this difference is not recognized.

The discussion so far has suggested that much of reality is arrived at by negotiation. This thesis was illustrated by materials presented on legal processes by Newman and medical processes by Balint. These processes are similar in that they appear to represent clear instances of the negotiation of reality. The instances are different in that the legal bargaining processes appear to be more open and accepted than the diagnostic process. In order to outline some of the dimensions of the negotiation process and to establish some of the limitations of the analyses by Newman and Balint, two excerpts of cases of bargaining will be discussed: the first is taken from an actual psychiatric "intake" interview, the second, from a fictional account of a defense lawyer's first interview with his client.

THE PROCESS OF NEGOTIATION

The psychiatric interview discussed is from the first interview in Gill, Newman, and Redlich (1954). The patient is a 34-year-old nurse who feels, as she says, "irritable, tense, depressed." She appears to be saying from the very beginning of the interview that the external situation in which she lives is the cause of her troubles. She focuses particularly on her husband's behavior. She says he is an alcoholic, is verbally abusive, and won't let her work. She feels that she is cooped up in the house all day with her two small children, but that when he is home at night (on the nights when he *is* at home), he will have nothing to do with her and the children. She intimates, in several ways, that he does not serve as a sexual companion. She has thought of divorce but has rejected it for various reasons (e.g., she is afraid she couldn't take proper care of the children, finance the baby sitters). She feels trapped.[8]

In the concluding paragraph of their description of this interview, Gill *et al.* give this summary:

> The patient, pushed by we know not what or why at the time (the children—somebody to talk to) comes for help apparently for what she thinks of as help with her external situation (her husband's behavior as she sees it). The therapist does not respond to this but seeks her role and how it is that she plays such a role. Listening to the recording it sounds as if the therapist is at first bored and disinterested and the patient defensive. He gets down to work and keeps asking, "What is it all about?" Then he becomes more interested and sympathetic and at the same time very active (participating) and demanding. *It sounds as if she keeps saying "This is the trouble." He says, "No! Tell me the trouble." She says, "This is it!" He says, "No, tell me," until the patient finally says, "Well I'll tell you." Then the therapist says, "Good! I'll help you* [p. 133; italics added].

From this summary, it is apparent that there is a close fit between Balint's idea of the negotiation of diagnosis through offers and responses and what took place in this psychiatric interview. It is difficult, however, to document the details. Most of the psychiatrist's responses, rejecting the patient's offers, do not appear in the written transcript, but they are fairly obvious as one listens to the recording. Two particular features of the psychiatrist's responses especially stand out: (1) the flatness of intonation in his responses to the patient's complaints about her external circumstances; and (2) the rapidity with which he introduces new topics, through questioning, when she is talking about her husband.

Some features of the psychiatrist's coaching are verbal, however:

T. 95: Has anything happened recently that makes it . . . you feel that . . . ah . . . you're sort of coming to the end of your rope? I mean I wondered what led you . . .
P. 95: (Interrupting.) It's nothing special. It's just everything in general.
T. 96: What led you to come to a . . .
P. 96: (Interrupting.) It's just that I . . .
T. 97: . . . a psychiatrist just now? [1]
P. 97: Because I felt that the older girl was getting tense as a result of . . . of my being stewed up all the time.
T. 98: Mmmhnn.
P. 98: Not having much patience with her.
T. 99: Mmmhnn. (Short Pause.) Mmm. And how had you imagined that a psychiatrist could help with this? (Short Pause.) [2]

---

[8]Since this interview is complex and subtle, the reader is invited to listen to it himself and compare his conclusions with those discussed here. The recorded interview is available on the first L.P. record that accompanies Gill, Newman, and Redlich (1954).

P. 99: Mmm . . . maybe I could sort of get straightened out . . . straighten things out in my own mind. I'm confused. Sometimes I can't remember things that I've done, whether I've done 'em or not or whether they happened.

T.100: What is it that you want to straighten out?

(Pause)

P.100: I think I seem mixed up.

T.101: Yeah? You see that, it seems to me, is something that we really should talk about because . . . ah . . . from a certain point of view somebody might say, "Well now, it's all very simple. She's unhappy and disturbed because her husband is behaving this way, and unless something can be done about that how could she expect to feel any other way." But, instead of that, you come to the psychiatrist, and you say that you think there's something about you that needs straightening out. [3] I don't quite get it. Can you explain that to me? (Short pause).

P.101: I sometimes wonder if I'm emotionally grown up.

T.102: By which you mean what?

P.102: When you're married you should have one mate. You shouldn't go around and look at other men.

T.103: You've been looking at other men?

P.103: I look at them, but that's all.

T.104: Mmmhnn. What you mean . . . you mean a grown-up person should accept the marital situation whatever it happens to be?

P.104: That was the way I was brought up. Yes.

(Sighs.)

T.105: You think that would be a sign of emotional maturity?

P.105: No.

T.106: No. So?

P.106: Well, if you rebel against the laws of society you have to take the consequences.

T.107: Yes?

P.107: And it's just that I . . . I'm not willing to take the consequences. I . . . I don't think it's worth it.

T.108: Mmhnn. So in the meantime then while you're in this very difficult situation, you find yourself reacting in a way that you don't like and that you think is . . . ah . . . damaging to your children and yourself? Now what can be done about that?

P.108: (Sniffs; sighs.) I dunno. That's why I came to see you.

T.109: Yes. I was just wondering what you had in mind. Did you think a psychiatrist could . . . ah . . . help you face this kind of a situation calmly and easily and maturely? [4] Is that it?

P.109: More or less. I need somebody to talk to who isn't emotionally involved with the family. I have a few friends, but I don't like to bore them. I don't think they should know . . . ah . . . all the intimate details of what goes on.

T.110: Yeah?

P.110: It becomes food for gossip.

T.111: Mmmhnn.

P.111: Besides they're in . . . they're emotionally involved because they're my friends. They tell me not to stand for it, but they don't understand that if I put my foot down it'll only get stepped on.

T.112: Yeah.

P.112: That he can make it miserable for me in other ways. . . .

T.113: Mmm.

P.113: . . . which he does.

T.114: Mmmhnn. In other words, you find yourself in a situation and don't know how to cope with it really.

P.114: I don't.

T.115: You'd like to be able to talk that through and come to understand it better and learn how to cope with it or deal with it in some way. Is that right?
P.115: I'd like to know how to deal with it more effectively.
T.116: Yeah. Does that mean you feel convinced that the way you're dealing with it now. . .
P.116: There's something wrong of course.
T.116: . . . something wrong with that. Mmmhnn.
P.117: There's something wrong with it [pp. 176–182].

Note that the therapist reminds her *four times*[9] in this short sequence that she has come to see a *psychiatrist*. Since the context of these reminders is one in which the patient is attributing her difficulties to an external situation, particularly her husband, it seems plausible to hear these reminders as subtle requests for analysis of her own contributions to her difficulties. This interpretation is supported by the therapist's subsequent remarks. When the patient once again describes external problems, the therapist tries the following tack:

T.125: I notice that you've used a number of psychiatric terms here and there. Were you specially interested in that in your training, or what?
P.125: Well, my great love is psychology.
T.126: Psychology?
P.126: Mmmhnn.
T.127: How much have you studied?
P.127: Oh (Sighs.) what you have in your nurse's training, and I've had general psych, child and adolescent psych, and the abnormal psych.
T.128: Mmmhnn. Well, tell me . . . ah . . . what would you say if you had to explain yourself what is the problem?
P.128: You don't diagnose yourself very well, at least I don't.
T.129: Well you can make a stab at it. (Pause) [pp. 186–187].

This therapeutic thrust is rewarded: the patient gives a long account of her early life which indicates a belief that she was not "adjusted" in the past. The interview continues:

T.135: And what conclusions do you draw from all this about why you're not adjusting now the way you think you should?
P.135: Well, I wasn't adjusted then. I feel that I've come a long way, but I don't think I'm still . . . I still don't feel that I'm adjusted.
T.136: And you don't regard your husband as being the difficulty? You think it lies within yourself?
P.136: Oh he's a difficulty all right, but I figure that even . . . ah . . . had . . . if it had been other things that . . . that this probably—this state— would've come on me.
T.137: Oh you do think so?
P.137: (Sighs.) I don't think he's the sole factor. No.
T.138: And what are the factors within. . .
P.138: I mean. . .
T.139: . . . yourself?
P.139: Oh it's probably remorse for the past, things I did.
T.140: Like what? (Pause.) It's sumping' hard to tell, hunh? (Short pause) [pp. 192–194].

[9]Numbers in brackets added.

After some parrying, the patient tells the therapist what he wants to hear. She feels guilty because she was pregnant by another man when her present husband proposed. She cries. The therapist tells the patient she needs and will get psychiatric help, and the interview ends, the patient still crying. The negotiational aspects of the process are clear: After the patient has spent most of the interview blaming her current difficulties on external circumstances, she tells the therapist a deep secret about which she feels intensely guilty. The patient, and not the husband, is at fault. The therapist's tone and manner change abruptly. From being bored, distant, and rejecting, he becomes warm and solicitous. Through a process of offers and responses, the therapist and patient have, by implication, negotiated a shared definition of the situation—the patient, not the husband, is responsible.

A CONTRASTING CASE

The negotiation process can, of course, proceed on the opposite premise, namely that the client is not responsible. An ideal example would be an interrogation of a client by a skilled defense lawyer. Unfortunately, we have been unable to locate a verbatim transcript of a defense lawyer's initial interview with his client. There is available, however, a fictional portrayal of such an interview, written by a man with extensive experience as defense lawyer, prosecutor, and judge. The excerpt to follow is taken from the novel, *Anatomy of a Murder* (Traver, 1959).

The defense lawyer, in his initial contact with his client, briefly questions him regarding his actions on the night of the killing. The client states that he discovered that the deceased, Barney Quill, had raped his wife; he then goes on to state that he then left his wife, found Quill, and shot him.

> "How long did you remain with your wife before you went to the hotel bar?"
> "I don't remember."
> "I think it is important, and I suggest you try."
> After a pause. "Maybe an hour."
> "Maybe more?"
> "Maybe."
> "Maybe less?"
> "Maybe."
>
> I paused and lit a cigar. I took my time. I had reached a point where a few wrong answers to a few right questions would leave me with a client—if I took his case—whose cause was legally defenseless. Either I stopped now and begged off and let some other lawyer worry over it or I asked him the few fatal questions and let him hang himself. Or else, like any smart lawyer, I went into the Lecture. I studied my man, who sat as inscrutable as an Arab, delicately fingering his Ming holder, daintily sipping his dark mustache. He apparently did not realize how close I had him to admitting that he was guilty of first degree murder, that is, that he "feloniously, willfully and of his malice afore-thought did kill and murder one Barney Quill." The man was a sitting duck [p. 43].

The lawyer here realizes that his line of questioning has come close to fixing the responsibility for the killing on his client. He therefore shifts his ground by beginning "the lecture":

The Lecture is an ancient device that lawyers use to coach their clients so that the client won't quite know he has been coached and his lawyer can still preserve the face-saving illusion that he hasn't done any coaching. For coaching clients, like robbing them, is not only frowned upon, it is downright unethical and bad, very bad. Hence the Lecture, an artful device as old as the law itself, and one used constantly by some of the nicest and most ethical lawyers in the land. "Who, me" I didn't tell him what to say," the lawyer can later comfort himself. "I merely explained the law, see." It is a good practice to scowl and shrug here and add virtuously: "That's my duty, isn't it?"

. . . "We will now explore the absorbing subject of legal justification or excuse," I said.

. . . "Well, take self-defense," I began. "That's the classic example of justifiable homicide. On the basis of what I've so far heard and read about your case I do not think we need pause too long over that. Do you?"

"Perhaps not," Lieutenant Manion conceded. "We'll pass it for now."

"Let's," I said dryly. "Then there's the defense of habitation, defense of property, and the defense of relatives or friends. Now there are more ramifications to these defenses than a dog has fleas, but we won't explore them now. I've already told you at length why I don't think you can invoke the possible defense of your wife. When you shot Quill her need for defense had passed. It's as simple as that."

"Go on," Lieutenant Manion said, frowning.

"Then there's the defense of a homicide committed to prevent a felony—say you're being robbed—; to prevent the escape of the felon—suppose he's getting away with your wallet—; or to arrest a felon—you've caught up with him and he's either trying to get away or has actually escaped.". . .

. . . "Go on, then; what are some of the other legal justifications or excuses?"

"Then there's the tricky and dubious defense of intoxication. Personally I've never seen it succeed. But since you were not drunk when you shot Quill we shall mercifully not dwell on that. Or were you?"

"I was cold sober. Please go on."

"Then finally there's the defense of insanity." I paused and spoke abruptly, airily: "Well, that just about winds it up." I arose as though making ready to leave.

"Tell me more."

"There is no more." I slowly paced up and down the room.

"I mean about this insanity."

"Oh, insanity," I said, elaborately surprised. It was like luring a trained seal with a herring. "Well, insanity, where proven, is a complete defense to murder. It does not legally justify the killing, like self-defense, say, but rather excuses it." The lecturer was hitting his stride. He was also on the home stretch. "Our law requires that a punishable killing—in fact, any crime—must be committed by a sapient human being, one capable, as the law insists, of distinguishing between right and wrong. If a man is insane, legally insane, the act of homicide may still be murder but the law excuses the perpetrator."

Lieutenant Manion was sitting erect now, very still and erect. "I see—and this—this perpetrator, what happens to him if he should—should be excused?"

"Under Michigan law—like that of many other states—if he is acquitted of murder on the grounds of insanity it is provided that he must be sent to a hospital for the criminally insane until he is pronounced sane.". . .

Then he looked at me. "Maybe," he said, "maybe I was insane.". . .

Thoughtfully: "Hm. . . . Why do you say that?"

"Well, I can't really say," he went on slowly. "I—I guess I blacked out. I can't remember a thing after I saw him standing behind the bar that night until I got back to my trailer."

"You mean—you mean you don't remember shooting him?" I shook my head in wonderment.

"Yes, that's what I mean."

"You don't even remember driving home?"

"No."

"You don't remember threatening Barney's bartender when he followed you outside after the shooting—as the newspaper says you did?" I paused and held my breath. "You don't remember telling him, 'Do you want some, too, Buster?'?"

The smoldering dark eyes flickered ever so little. "No, not a thing."

"My, my," I said blinking my eyes, contemplating the wonder of it all. "Maybe you've got something there."

The Lecture was over; I had told my man the law; and now he had told me things that might possibly invoke the defense of insanity. . . . [pp. 46–47, 57, 58–59, 60].

The negotiation is complete. The ostensibly shared definition of the situation established by the negotiation process is that the defendant was probably not responsible for his actions.

Let us now compare the two interviews. The major similarity between them is their negotiated character: They both take the form of a series of offers and responses that continue until an offer (a definition of the situation) is reached that is acceptable to both parties. The major difference between the transactions is that one, the psychotherapeutic interview, arrives at an assessment that the client is responsible; the other, the defense attorney's interview, reaches an assessment that the client was not at fault (i.e., not responsible). How can we account for this difference in outcome?

DISCUSSION

Obviously, given any two real cases of negotiation that have different outcomes, one may construct a reasonable argument that the difference is due to the differences between the cases—the finding of responsibility, in one case, and lack of responsibility, in the other, the only outcomes that are reasonably consonant with the facts of the respective cases. Without rejecting this argument, for the sake of discussion only, and without claiming any kind of proof or demonstration, I wish to present an alternative argument; that the difference in outcome is largely due to the differences in technique used by the interrogators. This argument will allow us to suggest some crucial dimensions of negotiation processes.

The first dimension, consciousness of the bargaining aspects of the transaction, has already been mentioned. In the psychotherapeutic interview, the negotiational nature of the transaction seems not to be articulated by either party. In the legal interview, however, certainly the lawyer, and perhaps to some extent the client as well, is aware of, and accepts the situation as one of striking a bargain, rather than as a relentless pursuit of the absolute facts of the matter.

The dimension of shared awareness that the definition of the situation is negotiable seems particularly crucial for assessments of responsibility. In both interviews, there is an agenda hidden from the client. In the psychotherapeutic interview, it is probably the psychiatric criteria for acceptance into treatment, the criterion of "insight." The psychotherapist has probably been trained to view patients with "insight into their illness" as favorable candidates for psychotherapy (i.e., patients who accept, or can be led to accept, the problems as internal, as part of their personality, rather than seeing them as caused by external conditions).

In the legal interview, the agenda that is unknown to the client is the legal structure of defenses or justifications for killing. In both the legal and psychiatric cases, the hidden agenda is not a simple one. Both involve fitting abstract and ambiguous criteria (insight, on the one hand, legal justification, on the other) to a richly specific, concrete case. In the legal interview, the lawyer almost immediately broaches this hidden agenda; he states clearly and concisely the major legal justifications for killing. In the psychiatric interview, the hidden agenda is never revealed. The patient's offers during most of the interview are rejected or ignored. In the last part of the interview, her last offer is accepted and she is told that she will be given treatment. In no case are the reasons for these actions articulated by either party.

The degree of shared awareness is related to a second dimension which concerns the format of the conversation. The legal interview began as an interrogation but was quickly shifted away from that format when the defense lawyer realized the direction in which the questioning was leading the client (i.e., toward a legally unambiguous admission of guilt). On the very brink of such an admission, the defense lawyer stopped asking questions and started, instead, to make statements. He listed the principle legal justifications for killing and, in response to the *client's* questions, gave an explanation of each of the justifications. This shift in format put the client, rather than the lawyer, in control of the crucial aspects of the negotiation. It is the client, not the lawyer, who is allowed to pose the questions, assess the answers for their relevance to his case, and most crucially, to determine himself the most advantageous tack to take. Control of the definition of the situation, the evocation of the events and intentions relevant to the assessment of the client's responsibility for the killing, was given to the client by the lawyer. The resulting client-controlled format of negotiation gives the client a double advantage. It not only allows the client the benefit of formulating his account of actions and intentions in their most favorable light, it also allows him to select, out of a diverse and ambiguous set of normative criteria concerning killing, that criteria which is most favorable to his own case.

Contrast the format of negotiation used by the psychotherapist. The form is consistently that of interrogation. The psychotherapist poses the questions; the patient answers. The psychotherapist then has the answers at his disposal. He may approve or disapprove, accept or reject, or merely ignore them. Throughout the entire interview, the psychotherapist is in complete control of the situation. Within this framework, the tactic that the psychotherapist uses is to reject the patient's ''offers'' that her husband is at fault, first by ignoring them, later, and ever more insistently, by leading her to define the situation as one in which she is at fault. In effect, what the therapist does is to reject her offers and to make his own counteroffers.

These remarks concerning the relationship between technique of interrogation and outcome suggest an approach to assessment of responsibility somewhat different from that usually followed. The common sense approach to interrogation is to ask how accurate and fair is the outcome. Both Newman's and Balint's analyses of negotiation raise this question. Both presuppose that there is an objective state of affairs that is independent of the technique of assessment. This is quite clear in Newman's discussion, as he continually refers to defendants who are "really" or "actually" guilty or innocent.[10] The situation is less clear in Balint's discussion, although occasionally he implies that certain patients are really physically healthy but psychologically distressed.

The type of analysis suggested by this chapter seeks to avoid such presuppositions. It can be argued that *independently* of the facts of the case, the technique of assessment plays a part in determining the outcome. In particular, one can avoid making assumptions about actual responsibility by utilizing a technique of textual criticism of a transaction. The key dimension in such work would be the relative power and authority of the participants in the situation.[11]

As an introduction to the way in which power differences between interactants shape the outcome of negotiations, let us take as an example an attorney in a trial dealing with "friendly" and "unfriendly" witnesses. A friendly witness is a person whose testimony will support the definition of the situation the attorney seeks to convey to the jury. With such a witness the attorney does not employ power but treats him as an equal. His questions to such a witness are open and allow the witness considerable freedom. The attorney may frame a question such as, "Could you tell us about your actions on the night of ——?"

The opposing attorney, however, interested in establishing his own version of the witness' behavior on the same night, would probably approach the task quite differently. He may say: "You felt angry and offended on the night of ——, didn't you?" The witness frequently will try to evade so direct a question with an answer like: "Actually, I had started to. . . ." The attorney quickly interrupts, addressing the judge: "Will the court order the witness to respond to the question, yes or no?" That is to say, the question posed by the opposing attorney is abrupt and direct. When the witness attempts to answer indirectly, and at length, the attorney quickly invokes the power of the court to coerce the witness to answer as he wishes, directly. The witness and the attorney are not equals in power; the attorney used the coercive power of the court to force the witness to answer in the manner desired.

---

[10]In his foreword, the editor of the series, Frank J. Remington, comments on one of the slips that occurs frequently, the "acquittal of the guilty," noting that this phrase is contradictory from the legal point of view. He goes on to say that Newman is well aware of this but uses the phrase as a convenience. Needless to say, both Remington's comments and mine can be correct: The phrase is used as a convenience, but it also reveals the author's presuppositions.

[11]Berger and Luckman also emphasize the role of power, but at the societal level. "The success of particular conceptual machineries is related to the power possessed by those who operate them. The confrontation of alternative symbolic universes implies a problem of power—which of the conflicting definitions of reality will be 'made to stick' in the society [p. 100]." Haley's (1959) discussions of control in psychotherapy are also relevant. See also by the same author, "The Power Tactics of Jesus Christ" (1969).

The attorney confronted by an "unfriendly" witness wishes to control the format of the interaction, so that he can retain control of the definition of the situation that is conveyed to the jury. It is much easier for him to neutralize an opposing definition of the situation if he retains control of the interrogation format in this manner. By allowing the unfriendly witness to respond only by "yes" or "no" to his own verbally conveyed account, he can suppress the ambient details of the opposing view that may sway the jury, and thus maintain an advantage for his definition over that of the witness.

In the psychiatric interview just discussed, the psychiatrist obviously does not invoke a third party to enforce his control of the interview. But he does use a device to impress the patient that she is not to be his equal in the interview, that is reminiscent of the attorney with an unfriendly witness. The device is to pose abrupt and direct questions to the patient's open-ended accounts, implying that the patient should answer briefly and directly; and, through that implication, the psychiatrist controls the whole transaction. Throughout most of the interview, the patient seeks to give detailed accounts of her behavior and her husband's, but the psychiatrist almost invariably counters with a direct and, to the patient, seemingly unrelated question.

The first instance of this procedure occurs at T. 6, the psychiatrist asking the patient, "what do you do?" She replies "I'm a nurse, but my husband won't let me work." Rather than responding to the last part of her answer, which would be expected in conversation between equals, the psychiatrist asks another question, changing the subject: "How old are you?" This pattern continues throughout most of the interview. The psychiatrist appears to be trying to teach the patient to follow his lead. After some 30 or 40 exchanges of this kind, the patient apparently learns her lesson; she cedes control of the transaction completely to the therapist, answering briefly and directly to direct questions and elaborating only on cue from the therapist. The therapist thus implements his control of the interview not by direct coercion but by subtle manipulation.

All of the foregoing discussion concerning shared awareness and the format of the negotiation suggests several propositions regarding control over the definition of the situation. The professional interrogator, whether lawyer or psychotherapist, can maintain control if the client cedes control to him because of his authority as an expert, because of his manipulative skill in the transaction, or merely because the interrogator controls access to something the client wants (e.g., treatment or a legal excuse). The propositions are:

1a. Shared awareness of the participants that the situation is one of negotiation. (The greater the shared awareness the more control the client gets over the resultant definition of the situation.)

1b. Explicitness of the agenda. (The more explicit the agenda of the transaction, the more control the client gets over the resulting definition of the situation.)

2a. Organization of the format of the transaction, offers and responses. (The party to a negotiation who responds, rather than the party who makes the offers, has relatively more power in controlling the resultant shared definition of the situation.)

2b. Counteroffers. (The responding party who makes counteroffers has relatively more power than the responding party who limits his response to merely accepting or rejecting the offers of the other party.)

2c. Directness of questions and answers. (The more direct the questions of the interrogator and the more direct the answers he demands and receives, the more control he has over the resultant definition of the situation.)

These concepts and hypotheses are only suggestive until such times as operational definitions can be developed. Although such terms as offers and responses seem to have an immediate applicability to most conversation, it is likely that a thorough and systematic analysis of any given conversation would show the need for clearly stated criteria of class inclusion and exclusion. Perhaps a good place for such research would be in the transactions for assessing responsibility previously discussed. Since some 90% of all criminal convictions in the United States are based on guilty pleas, the extent to which techniques of interrogation subtly influence outcomes would have immediate policy implication. There is considerable evidence that interrogation techniques influence the outcome of psychotherapeutic interviews also. Research in both of these areas would probably have implications for both the theory and practice of assessing responsibility.

CONCLUSION: NEGOTIATION IN
SOCIAL SCIENCE RESEARCH

More broadly, the application of the sociology of knowledge to the negotiation of reality has ramifications that may apply to all of social science. The interviewer in a survey or the experimenter in a social psychological experiment is also involved in a transaction with a client—the respondent or subject. Studies by Rosenthal (1966) and Friedman (1967) strongly suggest that the findings in such studies are negotiated, and influenced by the format of the study.[12] Rosenthal's review of bias in research suggests that such bias is produced by a pervasive and subtle process of interaction between the investigator and his source of data. Those errors that arise because of the investigator's influence over the subject (the kind of influence discussed in this chapter as arising out of power disparities in the process of negotiation) Rosenthal calls ''expectancy effects.'' In order for these errors to occur, there must be direct contact between the investigator and the subject.

A second kind of bias Rosenthal refers to as ''observer effects.'' These are errors of perception or reporting which do not require that the subject be influenced

---

[12]Friedman, reporting a series of studies of expectancy effects, seeks to put the results within a broad sociological framework.

by investigation. Rosenthal's review leads one to surmise that even with techniques that are completely nonobtrusive, observer error could be quite large.[13]

The occurrence of these two kinds of bias poses an interesting dilemma for the lawyer, psychiatrist, and social scientist. The investigator of human phenomena is usually interested in more than a sequence of events; he wants to know why the events occurred. Usually this quest for an explanation leads him to deal with the motivation of the persons involved. The lawyer, clinician, social psychologist, or survey researcher try to elicit motives directly by questioning the participants. But in the process of questioning, as previously suggested, he himself becomes involved in the process of negotiation, perhaps subtly influencing the informants through expectancy effects. A historian, on the other hand, may try to use documents and records to determine motives. He would certainly avoid expectancy effects in this way, but since he would not elicit motives directly, he may find it necessary to collect and interpret various kinds of evidence which are only indirectly related, at best, to determine motives of the participants. Thus, through his choice in the selection and interpretation of the indirect evidence, he may be as susceptible to error as the interrogator, survey researcher, or experimentalist—his error being due to observer effects, however, rather than expectancy effects.

The application of the ideas outlined here to social and psychological research need to be developed. The five propositions suggested may be used, for example, to estimate the validity of surveys using varying degrees of open-endedness in their interview format. If some technique could be developed which would yield an independent assessment of validity, it may be possible to demonstrate, as Aaron Cicourel has suggested, the more reliable the technique, the less valid the results.

The influence of the assessment itself on the phenomena to be assessed appears to be an ubiquitous process in human affairs, whether in ordinary daily life, the determination of responsibility in legal or clinical interrogation, or in most types of social science research. The sociology of knowledge perspective, which suggests that people go through their lives constructing reality, offers a framework within which the negotiation of reality can be seriously and constructively studied. This chapter suggests some of the avenues of the problem that may require further study. The prevalence of the problem in most areas of human concern recommends it to our attention as a substantial field of study, rather than as an issue that can be ignored or, alternatively, be taken as the proof that rigorous knowledge of social affairs is impossible.

[13]Critics of ''reactive techniques'' often disregard the problem of observer effects. See, for example, Webb, Campbell, Schwartz, Sechrest (1966).

The Stability of Deviant Behavior over Time: A Reassessment[1]

9

INTRODUCTION

LIKE Chapter 8, this chapter applies labeling concepts to a particular context. In this case, however, the context is not actual events but research findings. Earlier studies of the stability of deviant behavior over time seem to commit the psychologistic fallacy. That is, they assume an isolated individual with symptoms rather than considering issues such as who it is that is reacting to these symptoms and how the severity of the symptoms of those who come to official attention compare with the severity of those who do not.

The medical model of mental illness has come under attack along a broad front in psychiatry, psychology, and sociology. Among psychiatrists, Szasz (1961) and Laing (1967) are representative of those who would reject the entire medical model and its associated concepts. Psychologists, particularly those who base their work on learning theory, have developed a case against the medical model growing largely out of work in conditioning and behavior modification.[2] Sociologists such as Lemert (1951), Goffman (1961), and Scheff (1966) have pointed out that the medical model assumes an individual isolated from society and have sought to develop a theory in which labeling and the processes of social

---

[1]This chapter was written in collaboration with Eric Sundstrom. Acknowledgment is also made here to advice given by Paul Wuebben, who read an earlier draft.

[2]A convenient summary of the critique of the medical model from the point of view of learning theory can be found in Ullman and Krasner (1969).

interaction play a crucial role. Since the medical model is still the principal organizing concept in psychiatric thought, this controversy is of considerable importance for both theory and practice in the area of mental illness.

The difference in outlook between those who subscribe to the medical model and its critics is so extensive as to make resolution of the controversy somewhat difficult. Those who hold to the medical model consider mental illness an illness like any other, in that mental illnesses have a cause, course, lesion, symptom pattern, and treatment of choice. The critics object that these attributes of the model have never been demonstrated in a scientific manner but rest entirely on clinical impressions. Furthermore, those systematic studies that are conducted have, for the most part, not taken the controversy over the medical model into account in the design and execution of the research. For this reason, it has not been altogether clear what the overall weight of evidence is in the controversy, or how one would set about collecting evidence that would be decisive in supporting one side or the other.

The purpose of this chapter is to examine the evidence relating to a single aspect of the controversy over the medical model. In evaluating competing theories, the basic problem is to find at least one dimension along which the theories present diametrically opposed hypotheses and then to find all the evidence relative to this dimension. Such a procedure helps to ascertain the relative validity of the competing theories, even though one has available only a very narrow band of evidence. The resulting evaluation, although provisional, can still be useful in helping to determine contemporary strategies in research and public policy.

There is one dimension along which the medical model and the most extreme of its competitors, the theory of the societal reaction, radically diverge and for which a relevant body of evidence is readily available. The dimension concerns the stability of ''symptomatic behavior'' over time. An unstated, but nevertheless very strong, premise of the medical model is that the ''symptoms'' of mental illness are mere surface manifestations of an underlying pathology. According to the model, if the underlying pathology is not checked, the symptoms are very likely to continue unabated. To state the matter in medical terms, schizophrenia and most other psychiatric illnesses are usually malign processes that are not self-limiting.

A conflicting view is found in the theory of the societal reaction or labeling theory of deviance. From the point of view of labeling theory, ''symptoms of mental illness'' are seen as violations of residual social norms. These violations are posited to be products of situations, usually, rather than of personal predisposition. It is further hypothesized that these violations are usually *normalized*, and that when deviant acts are normalized, they are likely to be of transitory social significance (this volume, Chapter 4, pp. 63–64). Finally, the theory argues that the most important single cause of the stabilization of residual rulebreaking is *labeling* (i.e., those social processes that lead to the stigmatization and isolation of the rule-breaker). This view sees involuntary commitment and treatment as one part of the labeling process.

The two theories thus arrive at completely opposite conclusions for psychiatric practice. The medical model leads to the decision rule, "When in doubt, diagnose and treat" (in the interest of prevention), which from the point of view of the theory of the societal reaction is equivalent to the rule, "When in doubt, label." The opposite rule is reached if one follows labeling theory: "When in doubt, normalize" (in the interest of preventing the stabilization of otherwise transitory behavior).

There is a body of literature bearing on the question of the long-term stability of "symptomatic behavior." A thorough review of available studies in this area is found in the article "Stability of Deviant Behavior through Time" (Clarizio, 1968). Although the author avoids some of the assumptions of the medical model, he seems to take others as given. This chapter reassesses the studies he cites in an attempt to make them relevant for comparing the predictions of the medical model and labeling theory.

A word of warning needs to be prefaced, however. It is our judgment that the studies discussed here are faulty in some very fundamental ways, because almost all of them assume at least some of the basic premises of the medical model. The very use of the term *mental illness* is, we feel, obfuscating for research and most other purposes. Furthermore, most of the studies to be reviewed were not designed as a test of the hypotheses under discussion here. Any evaluation based on these studies is, therefore, at best provisional. We feel, however, that some evidence is better than none at all, and that it is possible to glean from these studies clues about the relative validity of the competing theories. We begin by discussing Clarizio's conclusions and their underlying assumptions.

ANALYSIS OF CLARIZIO'S REVIEW

From his review of longitudinal studies of psychiatric symptoms, Clarizio (1968) concludes that "change seems to characterize the course of problem behavior as much as or more than stability." His approach is based on findings from two types of studies: (1) Retrospective studies examine histories of both psychiatric and normal populations for pathological and/or traumatic histories. Predominance of problematic childhoods in currently deviant adults is considered evidence demonstrating the stability of their earlier misbehavior. (2) In follow-up studies, psychiatric subjects are evaluated initially, monitored over time, and later reevaluated in an effort to find how lasting the initial behavior actually was.

Clarizio's main conclusions from his analysis of these studies are that: (1) only certain types of disturbed children (i.e., children involved in specific kinds of rule-breaking) develop into career deviants; and (2) stability of deviant behavior depends on the nature of the behavior. "Normal problem behavior" seems to have a very high probability of being resolved with increasing age; most "clinical problems," such as acting out and antisocial behavior, however, end to become stable, often in more than one-half of the hospitalized cases.

Clarizio offers no hypotheses to explain *why* certain types of behavior tend to stabilize, and he suggests no criteria describing or delineating the deviance that stabilizes. He tries to avoid medical-model entrenched language by not introducing the concept of "symptom" in connection with deviance, thereby trying to avoid its implicit assumptions. When he speaks of "normal" problems and, variously, "severe clinical problems," he leaves unclear whether he sees the problems as situational or as endopsychic syndromes.

Speaking of *problems,* however, especially in terms of types, has implications that resemble those associated with medical language. In ordinary usage, the notion of a person with problems connotes an endopsychic problem. That is, a problem is not over when the deviant act is finished, but rather is something the person carries about within him. Clarizio thus appears to be making an oblique reference to individual-specific characteristics when he discusses types of children identifiable by their behavior. In a sense, his treatment of behavior types is closely related to the medical malfunction concept, because identifying characteristics have to be noncontext-bound. Clarizio, then, has avoided some of the medical framework but has not escaped it completely.

Another way of analyzing the evidence Clarizio cites could allow somewhat different conclusions. He neglects the sociological perspective; some insights about its applicability could be gained by seeing it in conjunction with these studies. This would support labeling theory if the evidence can be taken to show that labeling is associated with deviance stabilization. The medical model would find confirmation if some individual causal hypotheses could be show to hold.

Clarizio's first point is that "studies based on fairly typical (nonclinical) samples of children indicate that developmental problems are not particularly stable over time. . . ." Macfarlane, Allen, and Hanzik (1954) find that inter-age correlation of problems suggests nonpersistence. Lapouse and Monk (1964) "found age to be the variable most closely associated with the amount of behavior deviations, with young children surpassing older." These authors conclude that behavior deviations in children are age-bound events. Clarizio asserts that "in brief, studies based on nonpsychiatric populations indicate that behavior problems do not tend to be chronic. . . ." From the point of view of labeling theory, these results are interpreted to mean that nonpsychiatric populations have very good chances for experiencing denial rather than psychiatric labeling.

RETROSPECTIVE STUDIES

This type of study examines the history of a given group for behavior trends that may later be shown to be significant. Clarizio's citations include two approaches. In the first, backgrounds for psychiatric populations are compiled after the fact, with the intention of showing that some childhood experiences predispose subjects toward deviance as adults.

Kasanin and Veo (1932) obtained school histories for 54 hospitalized adult psychotics. Fifteen of the subjects (28%) were recalled by teachers as "peculiar and difficult." The teachers in this study knew of the subjects' status as "psychotic," so some bias is expected in their retrospective evaluations. It seems reasonable to assume that the teachers would tend to selectively remember details that are consistent with their present pictures of the subjects.

Bower, Shellhammer, Daily, and Bower (1960), however, controlled for rater bias by not revealing subjects' status and found "similar results," according to Clarizio. In the Bower study, the subjects who actually became schizophrenic were not perceived as unusual or disturbed by their teachers. Since only the very onset of schizophrenia was consistently recognized, ratings by teachers generally proved to have very little predictive value.

These findings are quite vague. Some adult deviants seem to have childhood histories of misbehavior—perhaps one-fourth, if Kasanin and Veo's study (1932) is indicative. Clarizio's other type of retrospective study dispels some of the confusion; here the authors examined healthy and abnormal populations as if they were trying to construct patterns explaining adult deviance and found about the same amount of traumatic histories for each group.

Renaud and Estes (1961) studied 100 mentally healthy adults and found that "their biographies do not differ appreciably, if at all, from those of psychiatric patients with respect to the amount of childhood experiences traditionally considered to prognose ineffective functioning and maladjustment." As the authors of this study observe, most personality development theories are at a loss to explain the dynamics of healthy adjustment. As a rule, pathologies and maladaptations receive most of the attention.

Schofield and Balian (1959) found that nearly one-fourth of 150 normal adults had "traumatic histories"; this is, coincidently, almost the same fraction of "peculiar and difficult" teacher ratings found by Kasanin and Veo (1932) for adult "psychotics." From these studies, it appears that healthy, exemplary adults seem about as likely to have traumatic histories as "mentally ill" ones. This evidence casts some doubt on the validity of applying developmental models of personality to the etiologies of mental illness.

FOLLOW-UP STUDIES

In these studies, which constitute the majority of Clarizio's citations, the sample populations are chosen and interviewed in advance. Then they are monitored and their case histories assembled over a period of time. This approach has the advantage of producing documented initial subject-ratings instead of depending on the memories of subjects and witnesses to reconstruct the initial states. The disadvantage of the approach is that follow-ups are based on clinical samples, which means that the subjects' behavior is invariably labeled at the outset. These studies, therefore, investigate only labeled behavior and cannot make reference to subjects who experienced normalization.

The focus of these studies is on symptoms (types of behavior) and their course over time. The main results were as follows:

1. Morris, Soroker, and Burrus (1954) found, in a 17–27-year follow-up of 54 childhood "internal reactors" (shy, withdrawn children), that about two-thirds achieved satisfactory adjustment, one-third marginal adjustment, and only one was rehospitalized. They concluded that introverted youngsters have a low probability of developing schizophrenia. In another study, based on a psychiatric sample, these authors found that extroverts and ambiverts tended to be rehospitalized more than introverts. Antisocial behavior was especially predictive.

2. Namche, Waring, and Ricks (1964) showed that childhood patients who were rehospitalized as adult schizophrenics also had histories characterized by theft, truancy, running away, and antisocial sexual activity.

3. Coolidge, Brodie, and Feeney (1964) demonstrated the transiency of school phobia; 47 of 49 phobics returned to school.

4. Balow and Blomquist (1965) found that severe childhood reading problems tended to resolve themselves over time. Most of their subjects were reading as adults.

5. Levitt, Beiser, and Robertson (1959) discovered that there was "no difference" (statistically) between treated and untreated subjects from a sample of 1006 guidance clinic patients. The course of neurotic symptoms proved independent of therapy (5 interviews or more), but the tendency was for the neuroses to be transitory.

6. Berkowitz (1955) found that three-fourths of patients who manifested pre-delinquent behavior as children grew up with no record of delinquency.

7. Eisenberg (1956) found stability in autistic behavior if the patient was mute by age five and transiency if useful speech was present. Three-fourths of childhood schizophrenics attained either marginal adjustment or were continuously institutionalized; only one-fourth achieved satisfactory adjustment.

THE ROBBINS' STUDY

All of the studies just cited utilize a similar follow-up approach; and their theoretical rationales have common points. The best known, most thorough, recent, and complete follow-up cited by Clarizio is Robbins' book, *Deviant Children Grown Up* (1966). Because Robbins' study represents the approach and makes explicit some of the underlying assumptions of the follow-up studies previously cited, it warrants a detailed examination. The same critique will apply equally to all similar follow-up studies.

Robbins (1966) asserts that knowing the natural history of a psychiatric syndrome helps in discovering its variations, the conditions from which it is likely to arise, and its course over time. Rather than postulate a single causal or predisposing factor, Robbins claims only that a restricted group of factors can be said to lead to a particular syndrome. Given this premise, she feels that "after it is established that a given set of symptoms identifies subjects who are and will remain homogeneous with respect to diagnosis, one can seek the common antecedents to this syndrome, antecedents which may eventually be shown to constitute its causes.''

Working from this theoretical position, Robbins proceeded to gather the psychiatric initial interview files for 524 patients seen at a St. Louis child guidance clinic between 1924 and 1929. One hundred control subjects, who had no psychiatric history at the time, were also chose. Through a process of interviewing relatives, employers, credit agencies, correction institutions, psychiatrists, and other witnesses, as well as the subjects themselves. Robbins was able to construct histories of the original syndromes 30 years later.

Robbins' special interest is the sociopathic personality, whose childhood misbehavior proves stable and durable over time. This "disease" occurred almost exclusively in boys referred to the clinic for antisocial behavior, especially theft. Some other childhood symptoms prognostic of sociopathy include incorrigibility, running away, discipline problems, aggressiveness, truancy, bad companions, etc. As adults, Robbins' "sociopaths" were operationally defined as having at least five antisocial symptoms from a specific list. Some of the most common ones were poor work history (85% of the sociopathic subjects), financial dependence (79%), marital problems (81%), multiple arrests (75%), and ever-incarcerated (73%).

It was found that 45% of the clinical group had five or more adult symptoms (from a list of over 20), as compared with 4% of the controls. Fifty-two percent of the control group were said to be free of adult psychiatric "disease," as against only 20% of the patients. A striking 34% of the patients had "seriously disabling symptoms," which corresponded to only 8% of the controls. These results were then to indicate that certain childhood symptoms, especially antisocial behavior, precede development of a sociopathic adult personality.

However, Robbins also found a somewhat different picture for neurotic symptoms other than hysteria. Not only were childhood neuroses useless as predictors of adult behavior, but the controls developed greater percentages of adult neurosis than did the clinical subjects. Thus, significant findings were limited exclusively to hysteria and sociopathy; neurotic behavior was simply too transient even to allow statistical inference.

Robbins clearly advocates the medical model and makes the assumptions appropriate to it as just discussed. Her adherence to the germ-theory analogy is striking. She speaks of "syndromes" as one would speak of contagious diseases; but in the case of deviance, it is certain *behavior*, not microorganisms, that she assumes to set the course of future pathology.

Robbins uses a categorization for rule-breaking behavior similar to Clarizio's, in which psychoses (and the internal ordered hierarchy of subdisorders) are more severe than the neuroses (assuming agreement on definitions and interpretations). Furthermore, she assumes that the severe cases will necessarily come to professional treatment, and that those cases which she did not investigate, could be false. If it is true that much deviance is denied, it is quite possible that Robbins dealt with only a fraction of rule-breaking behavior.

Robbins takes another fundamental point for granted: She assumes that her control group is comparable to her clinical sample. However, the two groups differ in the singularly important respect that the psychiatric patients all experienced labeling, while the controls operated under nonclinical conditions where denial is the prevalent mode. Hence, their normalized behavior cannot be carelessly thrown into the same analytic category with that of labeled ("sick") subjects. Also, according to labeling theory, conditions of symptom remission are not comparable; the labeled patient has tremendous barriers to overcome because he is covertly expected to continue misbehaving. Nonpatients are encouraged and rewarded for symptom remission, and the dynamics of their situation are favorable to resumption of normal behavior.

If the problem becomes discovering the differences between the probably-normalized behavior of controls and the clearly labeled deviances of clinic patient, Robbins' study can be seen as relevant. The evidence points out that careers in deviance are associated with labeling. While only 8% of the controls become sociopathic, 45% of the clinical population developed into career deviants. In addition to their psychiatric histories, over three-fourths of these adult sociopaths experienced juvenile court proceedings and the labeling intrinsic in that process.

CONCLUSION

Clarizio's conclusions from his assessment of studies of the stability of psychiatric symptoms lead one to question the medical model, since he reports that only in some cases do symptoms become stable. This chapter further emphasizes the lack of support for the medical model by pointing to some of the dubious assumptions Clarizio has accepted in those studies reporting stability. A central assumption made by Clarizio is that the symptoms of persons coming to the attention of clinics and hospitals are more "severe" than the symptoms of those who do not come to official attention. Labeling theory makes this assumption problematic by its interpretation that contingencies external to the rule-breaker more usually determine the societal reaction than the amount and extent of his rule-breaking. Given this alternative interpretation, all of the studies that to Clarizio indicate the stability of symptoms among psychiatric (labeled) populations instead support the hypotheses of labeling as a central cause for stabilization of deviant behavior. We suggest, therefore, that the available evidence indicates one of the crucial assumptions underlying application of the medical model to "mental illness" to be untenable. We suggest the need for longitudinal studies of labeled and unlabeled residual rule violation, set up specifically to test the relative predictive power of the medical model and labeling theory.

One of the authors has earlier suggested (Scheff, 1966:199) the outlines for a study of this kind, a field experiment: "In such a study, a survey would be used to locate rule-breakers who have not been labeled in the community. The rule-breakers would be divided into groups according to the degree and amount of their violations, with perhaps one group who repeatedly violated fundamental rules, at one extreme, and at the other, a group of persons who infrequently violated less important rules. Whatever the number and composition of these groups, each would be further divided at random into a labeled group and "normalization" group. That is, the rule-breakers in the labeled group would be exposed to the normal processes of recognition, definition, and treatment as mentally ill, and the denial group would be shielded from such processes. The effects of the labeling and normalization could then be systematically assessed over a period of time."

A field experiment of this type would require a considerable expenditure of time, money, and ingenuity to be carried out properly. It would also involve some ethical problems, since allowing some of the persons violating residual rules those in the denial group, to go without treatment, would be perceived as a breach of medical ethics by most psychiatrists. Even in the face of these difficulties, however, the crucial evidence that might result could be sufficiently significant to warrant serious consideration for this type of research.

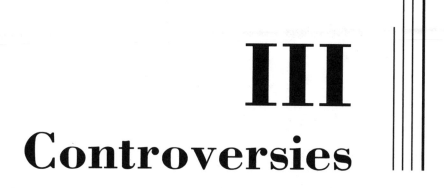

III

Controversies

On Reason and Sanity:
Some Political Implications
of Psychiatric Thought

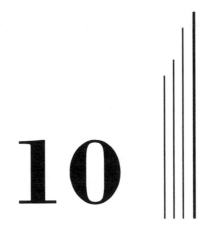

10

This chapter suggests that the established view of mental illness, the medical model, has implications that go far beyond the issues of diagnosis and treatment: the implications for global politics are discussed. Although this chapter was written during the Vietnam War, it still has contemporary relevance, since the Cold War continues to the present day.

About 75 years ago, a psychologist named Stratton conducted a series of excellent studies of the individual's perceptual world (1897a; 1987b). His procedure was unusual but simple: he designed a pair of prismatic spectacles which inverted his field of vision. He wore these glasses during all his waking hours for several periods of many weeks. One of his findings, as may be expected, was that the experience, at least initially, was almost totally disorienting. The inversion of up and down destroyed his customary world, so that even the most trivial kind of activity, such as tying his shoelaces, was well nigh impossible.

It can be argued that the individual's experience is mediated by a whole series of absolute dimensions, which give him a sense of continuity, mastery, and agency in his endeavors. Some of the dimensions are physical, such as up and down, left and right, the geographic sense of location in space, the temporal or historic sense of location in time (with respect to a calendar, say). Some of these axes are not physical but social and/or psychological. In a racist society, for example, the axis of racial separation is probably one such absolute dimension. Any perturbation along this axis is perceived by the members of the society as a cataclysmic dislocation, with the concomitant feelings of vertigo, nausea, and paralysis. The worth and value of a white man, his sense of self-esteem, in such a society, is constantly witnessed and affirmed by his sense of the inferiority of the black. The racial axis allows him to locate himself, not in physical time and space, but in social time and in moral space.

In an experiment somewhat analogous to Stratton's, a white man, Griffin, changed the color of his skin and became a "Negro" (1960). Like Stratton, he experienced almost total disorientation. An interesting difference between the two studies, however, was that Griffin's experience proved to be irreversible. He was thrown out of orbit, so to speak. When Stratton took off the glasses, he returned to his customary place in his society, an ordinary man among men. But Griffin's experiment so perturbed his position in the society that he found himself unable to return to his customary place.

In modern mass societies, there are probably many other important absolute axes, such as nationality and ideology. In the United States, particularly, the capitalist–communist axis and the closely related axis of nationalism, which separates Americans from aliens, probably operates in a way similar to the racial axis just discussed. All three of these axes are similar psychologically in that they identify an ingroup, the white American, "free enterprise" population, at the expense of outgroups, the blacks, the communists, and the aliens.

There is another, more subtle axis of contemporary experience, which because it is more pervasive is even more important than those already mentioned. This is the axis of reason and unreason, rationality and irrationality, or, most relevant to our discussion here, the related axis of sanity and insanity, which, in its most contemporary guise, is the axis of mental health and mental illness. In a richly detailed account, Foucault (1967) has shown how the successive concepts of madness in the last 400 years of European history paralleled and reflected the successive conceptions of reason. Although Foucault's narrative is labyrinthine, it gives a marvelously embroidered description of the relationship between the ethos and the handling of the "insane." For our present purposes, it makes the central point: conceptions and practices regarding insanity are intimately related to and influence contemporary sensibilities concerning reason and rationality.

In this chapter, I wish to make two points. First, that the dimension of mental health and mental illness is not an absolute fact of nature, like the physical directions of up and down, but a moral axis, like the social separation of whites and blacks. Second, that the confusion of the absolute and social bases of the distinction between sanity and insanity has political consequences. I first discuss the cultural arbitrariness of contemporary concepts of sanity and insanity.

Although most researchers in the area of mental illness speak with assurance about diagnostic entities such as schizophrenia, the scientific basis for these classifications remains obscure at best. For the major mental illness classifications, none of the components of the medical model has been demonstrated: cause, lesion, uniform and invariate symptoms, course, and treatment of choice. Studies of the reliability of psychiatric diagnosis show the levels to be low. Even at the theoretical level, there is little consensus about the nature of these diseases, *vide* the concepts of *schizophrenia* and *sociopathy.*

In the areas of positive mental health, the confusion is even more apparent. In a review of concepts of mental health, Jahoda (1958) found six competing concepts:

1. Mastery of the environment
2. Self-actualization
3. Self-esteem
4. Integration of self
5. Autonomy
6. Adequacy of perception of reality

The prospect of choosing between these six different criteria, as advanced by different experts, is disquieting enough. When one notes that some of the criteria may be contradictory (e.g., mastery of the environment as against self-actualization, and perception of reality as against autonomy) and that none has been operationally defined or investigated, one begins to perceive the state of chaos which characterizes the concept from a scientific point of view. It would appear that mental health is not a physical fact but a value choice about what kind of men we *should* be and what kinds of values should be encouraged in our society. Whether one selects a notion like *aggressive mastery of the environment,* traditionally a Western ideal, or the more inward turning goal like *self-actualization,* which is more akin to traditional ideals in the Orient, is not dictated by the natural order of stably reoccurring regularities in nature, but by human choice.

Just as mental health may be seen as a value choice as to how men should behave, so the symptoms of mental illness can be seen as value choices of how men should not behave. Thought and behavior that are taken to be correct in each culture are so taken for granted that the assumptions of propriety are largely invisible to its members. If one goes to the local cafeteria and butts in at the head of the line, there would be a reaction from those standing in line. If the intruder asked what the trouble was, he would be told, "First come, first served," or some such remark. Suppose, however, he continued in line and decided not to carry his own tray for his food but to place his food on the tray of the stranger behind him. He might be told that in this cafeteria, one carries one's own tray. More likely, feeling that "everybody knows" that, he might be eyed with suspicion and alarm. Continuing the example, suppose that after sitting down with the stranger, he notices some food on his plate that looks particularly tempting. He reaches across the table, spearing some of the food with his fork. This action, although it is no more than the violation of custom, would probably place the offender beyond the pale.

There are literally myriads of customs associated with each culture that "go without saying" to the point that violations leave the conforming member of the society baffled. His society has not prepared him for violations; they exist outside his vocabulary of motives. In speaking even simple sentences, there are thousands of understandings about proper grammar, syntax, pitch, loudness, rhythm, gesture, etc., that are part of any living language. The most elementary conversation is embedded in a whole network of understandings about comportment. For example, there is a conversational distance, neither too far, nor too close. When one speaks, one looks in certain directions: at the hearer's eyes or mouth, but not at his ear or forehead. Breaking so simple a custom results in the most violent kind of reaction. If one looks at another's ear, for example, during a conversation, the other will try to save the situation by moving his eyes into your line of vision. If you persist in looking at his ear, you can get the other to move around in a full circle. The result of shifting one's line of vision from the eyes to an ear, merely an angle of a few degrees, is enormous: The transaction is completely disrupted.

Although the reaction to violation of customs such as the ones discussed here is violent and complete, it must be remembered that these customs are largely conventions in a particular culture and as such are, for the most part, arbitrary and subject to change and transformation. They are not absolute, sacred, or immutable.

Foucault (1967) traces the confusion of values and science in modern psychiatry from its beginning in the nineteenth century:

> As positivism imposes itself upon medicine and psychiatry, this practice becomes more and more obscure, the psychiatrist's powers more and more miraculous, and the doctor–patient couple sinks deeper into a strange world. In the patient's eyes, the doctor becomes a thaumaturge; the authority he has borrowed from order, morality, and the family now seems to derive from himself; it is because he is a doctor that he is believed to possess these powers, and while Pinel, with Tuke, strongly asserted that his moral action was not necessarily linked to any scientific competence, it was thought, and by the patient first of all, that it was in the esotericism of his knowledge, in some almost daemonic secret of knowledge, that the doctor had found the power to unravel insanity [p. 220].

It need hardly be mentioned that the "order, morality, and the family" from which psychiatrists "borrowed" authority are the order, morality, and family structure of a particular society and, therefore, do not constitute absolute axes.

But in the everyday life of the members of the society, these axes are seen as absolute and, therefore, as sacred and immutable. In a study somewhat akin to those of Stratton and Griffin, Goffman (1961) wandered the halls of St. Elizabeth's hospital. Dressed shabbily, he was usually taken to be a patient. His statement gathers some of its impact from the reversal of the dimension of the sane and the insane. In his analysis he identifies with the patients; most of his narrative is from their point of view. Readers of *Asylums* report some of the reactions that occur when an axis that is assumed to be absolute is reversed: fear, fury, and awe.

From my own studies of commitment proceedings and subsequent confirmation of these studies by others, it would seem that the separation of the members of a society along the axis of sanity and insanity is largely a product of social rather than medical or scientific selection. Virtually all persons who are proposed by members of the community (or by public agencies such as the police) are accepted for treatment. The medical "examinations" which supposedly determine whether the candidate is sane or insane are, as a rule, peremptory and ritualistic. The actual goal in most of these examinations, and this includes the various diagnostic evaluations in the hospital also, seems not to be *whether* the candidate is mentally ill, but *which* mental illness he has.[1] Like the separation of blacks and whites, the sorting of the insane from the sane is primarily a social fact and not a fact of nature. Human beings have literally hundreds of physical attributes that are as visible as skin color (height, weight, attractiveness, etc). That skin color is the criterion of separation is a social choice rather than the inevitable product of physical processes that lie outside of human control, as upholders of racist societies would have us believe. Similarly, the segregation of the "mentally ill" is also a product of social choice rather than the ineluctable product of genetic, biochemical, or psychodynamic processes, as the upholders of the psychiatric status quo would have us believe.

Let us now turn to the so-called mental illnesses, such as schizophrenia. There are two major issues here. The first deals with the question of the existence of a behavioral system, an entity that is referred to as "schizophrenia." As indicated, the scientific basis for this label is unclear. The second point, to some degree, is independent of the first. Even if it were granted that there were such a system, would it necessarily follow that the energies of reasonable men be directed toward finding, analyzing, and changing such behavior? According to the concept of *schizophrenia* that is held by some psychiatrists, the attributes of schizophrenia are withdrawal, flatness of affect, thought disorder, language aberrations, and hallucinations or delusions. The schizophrenic is pictured, therefore, as a passive, inward-dwelling remote person who lacks interpersonal and other competences that other members of the society see as necessary to maintain or improve one's status in society.

[1]Mechanic (1962) reported that the two hospitals he studied (in California) accepted all patients. My own systematic studies of the rates of acceptance and the thoroughness of the psychiatric examinations were conducted in Wisconsin and reported in this volume. Independent replication of my findings, in California, is found in the report: *The Dilemma of Mental Commitments in California* (1967). As a result of these findings, a new law, which substantially changed commitment and other proceedings (the Lanterman–Petris–Short law), went into effect on June 1, 1969, in California.

It is interesting to note that reviewers of the first edition of *Being Mentally Ill* in England accept these findings, which they take to demonstrate the inferiority of American psychiatry. They seem to take for granted, without any evidence, that English hospitals are more discriminating and English psychiatric examinations more thorough. The evidence I collected in an English psychiatric hospital in London contradicts this assumption. As far as I could tell, the rates of acceptance and the level of thoroughness there were identical to those I reported in the United States. For my summary report see Scheff (1966:523–524).

Although these symptoms are stated in such a way as to suggest that they are in some way deviations from absolute and immutable standards, this is not necessarily the case. Withdrawal may be considered to be a violation of customary expectations about the degree of social and interpersonal distance that is held in the society, flatness of affect, a violation of expectations about expressive gestures. The language aberrations can obviously be seen as transgressions, not against the rules of nature but of language, which are, of course, arbitrary. What about thought disorder and hallucinations and delusions? It has already been suggested that there are culturally derived rules about propriety. Similarly, it is suggested that there are culture-bound rules about thought and about reality. To illustrate rules about reality, consider the effort Western parents go through to convince their children that dreams and nightmares are not real, but that disease germs are real. The child has seen and experienced nightmares and never seen germs. After some struggle, the parents convince him. But in some traditional societies, the scheme is reversed: The dreams are real, and the germs are not.

Not only are the expectations which lead to the absolute rejection of "schizophrenic symptoms" arbitrary; it may be argued that the evaluation of conventional sanity as desirable and "mental disease" (e.g., schizophrenia) as undesirable should be reversed. According to the conventional picture of schizophrenics, they would not have the competence or the motivation to napalm civilians, defoliate forests and rice crops, and to push the button that would destroy much of the world that we know. These activities are carried out by persons sane by conventional definition and encouraged, or at least not discouraged, by the great majority of the "sane" people in the society.

Senator Richard Russell of Georgia, was head of the Armed Services Committee of the Senate and one of the three or four most powerful men in the United States. He said: "If we have to start over again with another Adam and Eve, I want them to be Americans; and I want them on this continent and not in Europe." Senator Russell's liberty will not be removed because of that statement: His speech is coherent, there was no evidence of delusions or hallucinations, his affect was appropriate to his patriotic sentiments, and there was no indication of thought disorder. His calm willingness to see virtually all of the 3 billion people on earth sacrificed to his notion of patriotism does not raise questions about his sanity, as long as we continue to use conventional ideas about sanity. The current definitions of insanity leave men like Senator Russell at large and with the power to snuff out life on this planet.

As many of the current discussions regarding "preventive detention" make clear, there is often great difficulty in predicting the dangerousness of a person from his history, actions, or statements. Persons who make threatening statements often do not carry them out. On the other hand, persons without any violence in their record have, on occasion, become murderers. The prediction of dangerous actions from past behavior is not a highly developed science. Even granting this, however, surely Russell's statement must stand as one of the most threatening ever made. A society in which there were even a little prudence would surely take steps, such as "preventive detention," to see that a man with Russell's ideas and power not be allowed to continue in a position where he might help put an end to the human race.

Current definitions of insanity mobilize society to locate, segregate, and "treat" schizophrenics and other persons who are "out of touch with reality." Perhaps the time has come to consider the possibility that the reality that the so-called schizophrenics are out of touch with is so appalling that their view of the world may be more supportive to life than conventional reality.

I am not suggesting that Richard Russell is insane, but that the contemporary vision of sanity and reason is arbitrary and distorted. Current notions of psychiatry and mental health bring to the present crisis of human experience stereotypes of danger and threat that make us ill-equipped to respond. By mobilizing the energies and sensibilities of our society to act against schizophrenics while remaining silent about the erosion of reason of the respectable leaders and their followers in the larger society, psychiatric practice and research helps to condone the status quo.

The implicit support given the status quo by current psychiatric concepts and practice is especially important since the man in the street takes psychiatry to be a scientific enterprise. To the extent that practitioners and researchers in the field of mental illness argue and act as if mental illness is largely a technical, scientific issue rather than an area that is almost completely governed by moral values, they are functioning as accomplices to the current moral status quo. It is always tempting for the scientist to take the easiest way, which is to treat his job as exclusively concerned with means rather than ends. This bureaucratization of science demeans the scientist to a mere technician and induces him to avoid his responsibilities as an intellectual and citizen.

> To become worthy of his power the scientist will need to develop enough wisdom and humane understanding to recognize that the acquisition of knowledge is intricately interwoven with the pursuit of goals. It has often been pointed out that the nineteenth century slogan, "Survival of the fittest," begged the question because it did not state what fitness was for. Likewise, it is not possible to plan man's future without deciding beforehand what he should be fitted for, in other words, what human destiny ought to be—a decision loaded with ethical values. What is new is not necessarily good, and all changes, even those apparently the most desirable, are always fraught with unpredictable consequences. The scientist must beware of having to admit, like Captain Ahab in Melville's *Moby Dick*, "All my means are sane; my motives and objects mad" [Dubois, 1959:229–230].

I am also not suggesting that psychiatrists and other workers in the field of mental illness are more at fault than the rest of the society. It seems evident to me that as the United States has become committed to counterrevolutionary manipulation of the whole world, virtually all of the segments of American society fall into place, either by acts of commission or omission (Houghten, 1968). What Conor Cruise O'Brien has called the "counterrevolutionary subordination" of science and scholarship has been proceeding apace for the last 20 years. Many social scientists are directly involved in the planning of brutal and inhuman procedures to be used by the military (e.g., the ''population control'' programs in Vietnam). Other scholars, though not directly involved, approve the steps taken. Still others, and this includes most of the foremost scholars, conduct their work in such a way that objective scholarship is suborned to the interests of American power (Chomsky, 1969).

What I am suggesting is that researchers in the field of mental illness, to the extent that they follow contemporary social definitions of sanity and insanity, reason and unreason, without question or investigation, are helping to further confound the moral issues by giving laymen the impression, however subtly or unintentionally, that there is absolute scientific justification for the prevailing American world view. It is our responsibility as scholars and students of human behavior to make the hidden moral values in psychiatry and mental health visible, so that they can be made the subject of research and open public discussion. Only in this way will we have borne witness as scientists and scholars by contributing our knowledge of human affairs to the area of politics. With patience and ingenuity, it should be possible to make the invisible visible. The enterprise I have in mind is not a small one: to explore and help recreate current concepts first of sanity, and more broadly, of reason and rationality.

Medical Dominance:[1] Psychoactive Drugs and Mental Health Policy

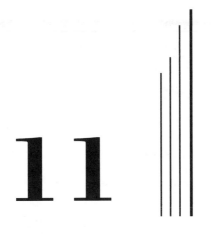

INTRODUCTION

THIS chapter concerns two highly interrelated issues: the benefits and risks of tranquilizers, on the one hand, and the issue of leadership in the mental health field, on the other. The two issues in practice are strongly connected, because psychiatrists, by law, overwhelmingly dominate the mental health field, and the treatment they use is tranquilizing medication. In 1974, when I wrote this chapter, the chief dangers I saw in the overuse of tranquilizers were physical side effects, like the irreversible brain damage caused by prolonged intake of thorazine, and sedation. At the present time, I believe that there is cause for even more concern about the possibility of the chemical suppression of distressful emotions in light of the enormously widespread prescription of tranquilizers like Valium. I find it hard to believe that these drugs are being used to correct metabolic errors, but instead that, they are used to mask negative feelings like fear and anxiety. If this is the case, we are facing a social problem of almost incalculable magnitude, a problem, like the moral dilemmas outlined in the last chapter, that is both cause and result of the established perspective on mental health and illness: the medical model.

The thesis of this chapter is that present mental health laws, which establish

[1]John Gai gave helpful advice, and Holly Seerley provided research assistance for this chapter. Leon Eisenberg and J. S. Hughes provided critical comments on an earlier draft.

medical dominance in the mental health field, are costly and probably unwise. These laws encourage treatment policies and practices which overemphasize chemotherapy and underemphasize sociopsychological treatment. Some of the scientific evidence relevant to these policies and practices is reviewed. The chapter ends with suggestions for alternative policies and for research projects that could provide support for legislative change.

Chemotherapy is the treatment of mental disorder that currently prevails in the United States. Particularly, for the more severe disorders, it has been established that tranquilizers and antidepressants are, in many cases, a quick, cheap, and effective way of stopping symptoms. Representing the opinion of the majority of psychiatrists is Eisenberg's (1973) statement: "Tranquilizers and anti-depressants are an effective chemotherapeutic means of managing acute psychotic disorders."

Chemotherapy not only has had practical results but also has suggested paths toward the theoretical understanding of the mechanisms of psychiatric symptoms such as hallucinations and delusions. Research on the biochemistry of the brain has suggested that symptoms of mental disorder may be caused by metabolic errors in the transmission of neural signals. It is hypothesized that these errors are corrected by the action of the tranquilizing drugs. Although these findings are suggestive, they are still inconclusive (Snyder, Banerjee, Yamamura, and Greenburg, 1974).

In light of these dramatic developments, the enthusiasm for chemotherapy that exists in the medical profession is understandable. What is more difficult to understand is why this enthusiasm has been allowed to prevail with so little examination of its short- and long-term effects. Although the benefits of the tranquilizers have been demonstrated exhaustively, there have been relatively few studies of the costs and risks associated with their use.

THE SOCIAL VALUE OF PSYCHOACTIVE DRUGS

Although chemotherapy has brought many benefits, it is conceivable, given what we already know, that an examination of the entire structure of the medical use of psychoactive drugs would show that the risks and costs outweigh the benefits. In terms of social policy, it is important not only to establish that chemotherapy is sometimes effective and that through research it could advance our understanding of some forms of mental illness, but also to establish the ratio of benefits to costs and risks over the whole spectrum of chemotherapeutic practice.[2] In order to make such an assessment, we need to know the answers to the following questions: First, in the entire population that is treated, what is the proportion of cases in which the treatment is effective and necessary? This is the question that controlled longitudinal studies are designed to answer. Second,

---

[2]A valuable discussion of the social implications of psychoactive drugs can be found in Lennard Epstein, Bernstein, and Ransom (1974).

what are the undesirable side effects of treatment, and in what proportion of the treated patients do they occur?

In assessing the value of a treatment in terms of social policy, these two questions of efficacy and of side effects are interrelated. At the other extreme, there are valueless treatments whose rate of efficacy is low and whose side effects are frequent and severe. As we shall see in the discussion following, the various forms of chemotherapy would appear to fall somewhere between these two extremes, with the phenothiazines (in the treatment of acute psychosis) and lithium carbonate closer to the positive value end of the continuum, the antidepressants of lesser value, and the phenothiazines in the treatment of chronic psychosis and the antianxiety drugs worse than useless.

The most dramatic changes in the field of mental health in recent years have been brought about in part by the use of thorazine (generic name: chlorpromazine) in the treatment of schizophrenia. Treatment with this drug played a major role in the great reduction of the patient population in mental hospitals that has been occurring since the early 1950s. Thorazine, like the other drugs of its type, the phenothiazines, appears to have distinctly antipsychotic properties; that is, the phenothiazines do not merely sedate but also interfere with the production of psychotic symptoms, at least in some cases.

It should be clear, however, that these drugs do not cure the disease; they merely stop the symptoms. Eisenberg (1973:120–121) writes: "Extensive clinical research has documented the effectiveness of the phenothiazines in terminating an episode of schizophrenia. The natural history of the disorder, however, indicates a substantial risk of recurrence and little residue of benefit from prior treatment."

Furthermore, the studies that show the efficacy of the phenothiazines for some patients also make clear that they are not effective for others. Using the avoidance of rehospitalization within 1 year as the criteria, controlled studies show that 60–70% of patients with diagnosis of acute schizophrenia on no drugs are readmitted within 1 year, while only 20–30% of patients receiving drugs are rehospitalized. Clearly, some 40% of the patients on drugs are helped to stay out of the hospital by the drugs, but 20–30% are not, and 30–40% of the patients in the study who did not receive drugs also avoided rehospitalization (Prien and Klett, 1972: 64).

Not all the controlled studies show even this much positive effect. In particular, several studies show that the difference between treated and placebo patients declines with the passage of time if intervals greater than 1 year are used. One study indicated that the differences may be as low as 10–15% after several years (Engelhardt, Rosen, and Freedman, 1967).

In one recent study, the passage of time causes the situation to be reversed. The adjustment of the placebo patients becomes significantly better than those who received the drugs. This study, by Rappaport (1974: 39, 138) concerns 120 first-admission, young, male patients diagnosed as schizophrenic. Comparisons were made on improvement in drug and placebo patients at two points in time:

after discharge from the hospital and at follow-up, which took place up to 3 years after discharge. Results are indicated in Table 11.1.

As can be seen from the table, a substantially larger proportion of the patients on drugs had improved at time of discharge compared with the placebo group. However, by the time of follow-up within 3 years, the situation was reversed; it was the placebo group that had a much larger proportion of improved cases. This study suggests, at least for a majority of these types of patients, that phenothiazines are not only ineffective but should not be used. This finding, which is in such stark contrast to existing medical belief and practice, requires some discussion.

Current practice with cases diagnosed as schizophrenia is to routinely administer phenothiazines. Most physicians believe that these drugs are usually effective. One basis for this belief is the large number of studies which suggest that the condition of patients being maintained on phenothiazines deteriorates when the drugs are removed. However, Tobias and MacDonald (1974), in their review of 40 such studies, (25 of which were uncontrolled and 15 controlled), conclude that because of methodological flaws, no inferences can be drawn. It would seem that further long-term studies of the type conducted by Rappaport are urgently needed. In summary, the evidence concerning the phenothiazines suggests that the drugs are effective in some cases, especially in the beginning of treatment, not effective in others, and actually harmful in others. We will now turn to the examination of the ways in which these drugs may do harm.

From the beginning of the use of these tranquilizers, it was known that they sometimes produced detrimental physical side effects:

> sedation and symptoms resembling Parkinson's disease are a problem for some patients and serious toxicity (persistent rhythmical involuntary movements of tongue and face, abnormal pigmentation, low white-cell count and jaundice) afflicts a substantial minority [Eisenberg, 1973: 24].

Eisenberg's estimate of the dangers of the side effects of the phenothiazines, like most psychiatric opinion, is probably understated. It would appear that a new syndrome of central nervous system disorder, tardive dyskinesia, has been created by phenothiazine use. According to Crane (1973: 126–127) its manifestations are

> slow, rhythmical movements in the region of the mouth, with protrusion of the tongue, smacking of the lips, blowing of the cheeks, and side-to-side movements of the chin, as well as other bizarre muscular activity. More careful examinations of patients on long-term drug therapy revealed that, not only the mouth, but practically all parts of the body could exhibit motor disorders, such as myoclonia, chorea, and athetosis. Overextension of the spine and neck, shifting of weight from foot to foot, and other abnormal postures indicated that the coordination of the various segments of the axial musculature was also affected. Less frequently, the syndrome resembled in every respect known neurological diseases, such as Huntington's disease, dystonia musculorum deformans, and postencephalitic brain damage.

TABLE 11.1   Evaluation of Patients by Time and by Treatment[a]

Patient's condition	At time of discharge (N = 120)		At follow-up (N = 75)	
	Drug	Placebo	Drug	Placebo
Better	40(78%)	39(57%)	21(57%)	30(79%)
Worse	11(22)	30(43)	16(43)	8(21)
Total	51	69	37	38

[a]Adapted from Rappaport (1974).

For patients on "maintenance" doses (i.e., long-term treatment), Baldessarini and Lipinski (1973) estimated that this reaction occurs in from 3 to 40% of the cases, with a mean of about 15%, a not inconsiderble group.[3] In the more severe reactions, the syndrome continues after the drug is removed. Like lobotomy, the phenothiazines may cause permanent, irreversible brain damage (see Crane, 1973: 127). The manufacturers also warn that these drugs have had many other side effects including "sudden, unexpected and unexplained death." This range of severe physical effects suggests that in some instances phenothiazine treatment may be worse than the disease it is supposed to cure.

Of perhaps equal significance are the psychological and social side effects of these drugs. Although it is difficult to make a clear assessment because of inadequate and conflicting evidence, most psychiatrists think that part of the effect of thorazine is sedation. For example, Allan (1975) writes: "thorazine is often used as a drug of choice because of the sedation it provides. This can be extremely beneficial in calming the patient, and is distinct from the anti-psychotic properties of the drug."

On the other hand, Crane (1973: 125), who is perhaps the leading authority on the physical side effects of the phenothiazines seems to disagree:

> Neuroleptics may reduce overactivity and belligerent behavior, but these are secondary effects of a general lessening of psychopathology. Sedation occurs only in the early stages of drug therapy in certain susceptible individuals, or when excessive doses are administered, particularly of chlorpromazine (thorazine).

A review of studies of the effect of thorazine on learning seems to bear out Allan's position rather than Crane's. Hartlage (1965:235) reports as follows: "Results of studies involving a number of animals, normal subjects, and psy-

---

[3]In a recent study, Crane found 51% of the patients in his sample suffering from physical side effects. The wide variation is probably due to variations in dosage levels, duration of treatment, and age of the groups studied.

chiatric patients tend to show significant declines in learning on a wide range of tasks, with a linear decline in learning with increased dosage levels.''

The social effects of the phenothiazines are virtually unknown. In a pioneering study, which still has not been replicated, Lennard, Epstein and Katzung (1967) administered a small dose of thorazine to one member of each of seven three-person discussion groups. He found a decrease of initiation of activity by the drugged member as against the placebos and, significantly, a consistent decrease of communications addressed to that person by the others. These findings are particularly significant because of the low dosage level, only 50 mg of thorazine. Since the average dosage of phenothiazines is considerably higher than this (1600 mg per day is not uncommon), and since Hartlage has suggested that decreases in learning are a linear function of increasing dosage, Lennard *et al.'s* (1967) findings are extremely important.

For our purposes, perhaps the most significant study of chemotherapeutic practice yet reported was done by Crane (1974), who determined the amount of overdosing and the physical side effects in a group of 160 long-term mental hospital patients. He first established a baseline behavior for each patient at the original drug level, whose drug levels ranged from 21 patients who were not on drugs to 17 who were getting between 700 and 1800 mg per day, CPZ, eq. (chlorpromazine equivalent: the amount of chlorpromazine that it would take to produce the effect of one of the other phenothiazines). Using this method, he was able to drastically reduce the dosage levels of all of the patients, including 28 patients that he removed from drugs entirely over the course of 1 year.

Over the course of a 3-year period, he reduced the drug level even more, from an average dose of 336 CPZ eq. to 134. On the basis of this study, it would appear that overdosing is a common occurrence since all of these patients had been overdosed for years, with a sizeable proportion of them overdosed by extremely large amounts (33% of these patients had been overdosed by 400 or more CPZ eq. a day).

Crane also determined that in this group of 160 patients, 81 (51%) had long-lasting physical side effects as a result of the drugs. In this group of 81 patients, he reduced the drugs to below the level that would cause side effects and still maintained the baseline behavior in all but 15% of the cases. In other words, in 85% of the cases, the physical damage that the drugs caused to the patients was completely unnecessary. Since Crane made no assessment of the social and psychological side effects, we cannot obtain a complete picture of damage caused by the drugs. If we think of this study in terms of Lennard *et al.'s* (1967) findings, we can see that in Crane's 3-year study, the average overdose was 202 CPZ eq., or approximately four times as great as the dose Lennard *et al.* used. We might, therefore, conjecture that there was considerable damage done to the social competence of the patients in this study. A similar estimate is possible following from Hartlage's report on the effect of chlorpromazine on learning. Since he suggested that decrement in learning is a linear function of level of overdose, it is not unreasonable to conclude that these patients probably suffered considerable psychological damage from the drugs.

What seems to be needed are long-term controlled studies of the efficacy of phenothiazines, which include consideration of both benefits and costs in the same study (i.e., these studies should include assessment of physical, psychological, and social side effects in both treated and placebo groups). Although there have been some 10,000 papers written on thorazine alone, not a single one of them has considered this issue. Until such studies are done, one is unable to demonstrate that the benefits of phenothiazine treatment outweigh the costs and risks.

Similar comments apply to the other major psychoactive drugs, the antidepressants and lithium carbonate, which are used for the treatment of depression and of manic-depressive psychosis, respectively. As in the case of phenothiazines, existing studies demonstrate that these drugs are effective in some cases, ineffective in others, and harmful in others.[4] Without further studies that include consideration of physical, social, and psychological side effects, one cannot accurately assess their value to society.

In the case of the antianxiety drugs, the picture is still less positive. The case of meprobamate is instructive. This drug, known as Miltown, was introduced in the late 1950s as an antianxiety tranquilizer. After many years and millions of prescriptions, it became clear in controlled studies that the drug could not be shown to have any more effect than placebos, and clinical experience indicated that the drug was addictive (see Greenblatt and Shader, 1971). For these reasons, meprobamate has been quietly withdrawn from use. In its place have come a number of other antianxiety tranquilizers, the best-known of which are Valium and Librium. Once again, however, history may be repeating itself—it now seems possible that Valium and Librium cannot be shown to have any effect greater than a placebo, and that they can be addictive.[5] Nyswander (1975:152–153) a psychiatrist well known for her studies of addiction, has warned that sustained use of Valium in large doses brings about "a far worse addiction than heroin, morphine, or demerol."

The history of the use of meprobamate, Valium, and Librium, when considered in the context of the histories of earlier psychiatric innovations such as lobotomy and electroconvulsive therapy, does not suggest a particularly optimistic outcome. I am not suggesting, of course, that chemotherapy has no value at all. As has already been stated, the effectiveness of phenothiazines and lithium carbonate for some cases of mental illness has been clearly established as well as the promise of advances in the understanding of the neurological bases of these

[4]For a review of studies, see Morris and Beck (1974), Prien and Caffey (1974). Physical side effects of lithium are listed in O'Connell (1974). Psychological damage done by lithium is noted in Aminoff, Marshall and Smith (1974).

[5]For strong doubts expressed about the efficacy of Valium and Librium by a consumer testing organization, see Consumer Reports (1974) and Gordon (1974).

types of mental illness. But the total costs and risks of chemotherapy, in the context of the medical practice in which it is based, may be unacceptably great, as indicated in the foregoing discussion.

One area where considerably more research on tranquilizer effects is urgently needed concerns dosage levels and psychological and social effects of drugs. Drug manufacturers acknowledge that there is sedation of some patients even at optimum-dosage levels. This problem is greatly magnified in cases where the dosage level is too high. The patient's reaction time, visual and verbal acuity, and social responsiveness are affected. I suspect, however, that there is great temptation for the physician to err toward overdose rather than underdose.

There is wide variation in patients' responses to tranquilizers—so much so that getting exactly the right dosage takes considerable time, observation of and consultation with the patient. In institutional practice, especially, the physician is likely to see an underdose as the more costly error, as the symptoms of the illness often recur as if there were no medication at all. Studies of the dosage levels in actual patient populations and of the social and psychological costs of the side effects at these levels would be useful in assessing the long-range social implications of current treatment policies.

SOCIAL–PSYCHOLOGICAL THERAPIES

Given the formidable side effects of chemotherapy, why is it there is so much unqualified enthusiasm by physicians? One reason is suggested by the foregoing discussion: The benefits of chemotherapy are often quickly apparent: cessation of the dramatic symptoms of acute psychosis. The costs, however, are less obvious: subtle lowering of competence, the possible masking of significant psychological or social conflict, or physical side effects which may be missed or confused with symptoms of the "illness."

Equally important are the weaknesses that physicians attribute to the forms of treatment alternative to chemotherapy, the various forms of sociopsychological therapy. Although there is a very large number of differing approaches, all of these forms of therapy contain, in varying proportions, the following elements (suggested by Mendel and Green, 1967:30-31):

1. The development of trust between patient and therapist(s)
2. Reflection of patient's thoughts, perceptions, and behaviors by the therapists to the patient: "This is how we see you"; supportive therapies emphasize this phase
3. Exploration of the history of the patient's thoughts, perceptions, and behaviors; expressive therapies emphasize this phase
4. Exploration of alternative ways of handling problems
5. Trial of alternative ways of handling problems

Encounter and Rogerian therapies emphasize the second phase, reflection. Psychoanalysis and the cathartic therapies stress the third phase, exploration of the patient's history. Behavior modification focuses almost exclusively on the fourth and fifth phases, trials of new behaviors. (Actually, all sociopsychological therapies, whatever their emphasis, are also dependent on the first phase, the establishment of trust.) Supportive therapies, when used in mental hospitals for prolonged and severe mental disorder, should contain all five elements.

I survey these phases of sociopsychological treatment to underscore the kind of detailed knowledge and understanding the therapist(s) must have of the patient: the minute particulars of the patient's existence and how these particulars are related to the patient's problems. Most physicians, given their extensive caseloads, see sociopsychological methods as impractical. They are seen as impossibly expensive, time-consuming, protracted, and of uncertain effectiveness. Given the choice between chemotherapy and sociopsychological methods, most physicians rely almost exclusively on chemotherapy.

Because chemotherapy does not remove the source of the disorder, there is a strong temptation for the psychiatrist to resort to continuous drugging, the so-called "maintenance therapy." Apparently, the majority of patients in mental hospitals and a sizeable proportion of the elderly in nursing homes are on high and continuous drug medication. Perhaps the most powerful of the drugs used for this purpose is Prolixin, a phenothiazine derivative. This drug is used in a long-acting form, with injections whose actions last for 2 weeks. Although commonly called "the magic elixir" among psychiatrists, it may be serving, at least in some cases, as a chemical straitjacket.

Since certain knowledge of the causation of mental disorder is virtually nil, the most prudent course of action, it seems to me, would be a treatment policy which combines the strengths of both methods, excluding neither. This policy is recommended by Mendel. He acknowledges (1975:121) that drugs can play a useful part in psychiatric therapy but has strong reservations about relying on them exclusively and urges restraint in the use of drugs:

> When the therapist delays the administration of drugs until the second outpatient visit or until the second day of crisis intervention, the amount of medication needed may be decreased by as much as 70 percent.

> To administer as little medication as possible is not only of value from an economic point of view and from a physiological point of view in terms of avoiding unnecessary side effects; one must also remember that the psychological factors too, can be antitherapeutic. The administration of medication may further reinforce feelings of helplessness and passivity in the patient.

The studies suggested in this chapter so far have concerned the relative costs and benefits of present treatment policy, which is oriented for the most part to chemotherapy. A much broader question concerns the costs and benefits of sociopsychological treatments and their relationship to chemotherapy. What are the pressures on therapists which induce them to rely so completely upon chemotherapy with its risks and uncertainties? Why are the sociopsychological treatments seen as so expensive and unreliable? To begin to answer these questions, it is useful to examine some questions of legal and administrative policy.

MENTAL HEALTH AND THE LAW

Present mental health laws and policy establish medical dominance by fiat. Medical dominance is not based on the competitive position of psychiatrists relative to other physicians, mental health professionals, and laymen in an open market of ideas and practices. The dominance of psychiatrists is largely a result of legal and social definitions. Although the status of mental disorder as a disease is uncertain from a scientific point of view, there is a consensus among most laymen and policymakers that mental disorder is in fact a disease and that psychiatrists, therefore, are necessary to control treatment.

Freidson (1970: xi) has argued that administrative and economic dominance of the professions, particularly that of medicine, lies at the root of all health-care problems: "professional dominance is the analytic key to the present inadequacy of the health services." For the reasons I indicate, in the following section, Freidson's argument applies especially strongly to the mental health field.

In mental hospitals, clinics, and psychiatric units of general hospitals, the present statutes require that psychiatrists must be not only on the staff, but that they must be in dominant positions. The law invests psychiatrists with authority on the basis of their training, which presumably makes them experts in the treatment of mental illness. However, these legal requirements are costly and wasteful. It is true that some of the tasks involved in therapy, principally the use of drugs, are related to the psychiatrists' training. Most of the tasks are not. That is, much of the function of leadership concerns administrative, psychological, and interpersonal issues. Most of a physician's training not only does not prepare him or her for these tasks, it also interferes in many ways. The bulk of a doctor's training concerns internal bodily states, which deflects interest and attention from the social and psychological concerns that loom so large in a psychiatric unit. Most of the physician's 9 years of training is wasted in this context. A social worker with 2 years of training is much less costly and usually has more training in administrative, psychological, and interpersonal processes.

The scarcity of physicians is another problem, indicated in part by the presence of a quite sizeable group of foreign-trained physicians in U.S. medical practice. About half the physicians licensed in 1975 belong to this group (Mick, 1975). Torrey and Taylor (1972) have argued that foreign-trained psychiatrists tend to be less qualified than those who received their training in this country. Certainly, the administrative and interpersonal tasks that psychiatrists face would be crucially affected by differences in competence in the English language and in cultural background. As an example, I cite the current practice in Texas of employing Cuban psychiatrists whose familiarity with English is, at best, rather weak.

As to the effectiveness of therapy, the legal requirement of medical control is also disruptive. Since psychiatrists are expensive and in short supply, the law guarantees that the therapist with the least contact and knowledge of the patients' condition will be the only staff member with authority for care. In most mental hospitals, the psychiatrist, who is responsible for treatment and vital decisions as to the patient's fate, such as admission and release, is apt to have a very large number of patients under his or her care, in some cases hundreds. The psychiatrist cannot possibly get the extended contact and detailed knowledge that would be involved in high-quality treatment. The law literally forces him or her to become a dispenser of tranquilizers with large numbers of patients. The psychiatrist cannot even do this well since he or she is apt not to obtain the detailed knowledge of the patients' conditions that should govern indications for use, side effects, and dosage regulation.

Furthermore, medical control is disruptive of cooperation among treatment staff. Since psychiatrists are scarce, most of the treatment staff will not be physicians but social workers, psychologists, nurses, and aides. In many cases, the most capable therapist or administrator in the group will not be the psychiatrist but a member of one of the other occupational groups. The arbitrary imposition of medical leadership by legal fiat stifles initiative and creates tensions and resentments which interfere with staff morale and, therefore, with therapeutic effectiveness.

I have noticed a second consequence of medical control which grows out of social modeling. The psychiatrist is the most prestigious and powerful person on the staff; thus, many of the staff members model their behavior on his or her behavior. Since the psychiatrist is also the person who has the least time for patients, it is not unusual to find many staff members in mental health units acting as if they had virtually no time to give to patients—social workers concentrating on the patients' family, psychologists on tests, nurses on records, and aides on house-cleaning—so the patients are left to their own devices.

The team concept of psychiatric treatment seems to me to be a feasible way out of this morass. A change in legal requirements is all that would be needed. I am not suggesting that psychiatrists be excluded from the treatment of mental illness, but only that they should not arbitrarily be designated as leaders. In the team concept, the leader of the group would be elected. A committee system in which there were representatives of the major groups, the psychiatrists, other professionals, the aides, and the patients would probably work best. The director of the unit would be elected from this committee. He or she may or may not be a psychiatrist. In this arrangement, medical skills would still be available; the psychiatrist, even if not the leader, would still be a part of the treatment team. In those cases, psychiatrists could probably use their best skills to greater advantage. For example, a psychiatrist relieved of administrative and psychotherapeutic duties may have the time to do a skillful job of drug therapy on a consultative basis.

It seems likely that a committee system would result in more effective leadership, because it would more efficiently utilize all of the skills present among members of the staff and lead to improvement of staff morale. Under these conditions, it is possible to envision psychiatric units which would be therapeutic communities: a realistic treatment plan would be rapidly developed for each patient, and there would be sufficient staff–patient contact such that effective therapy could occur.

The kind of research needed to evaluate the cost-effectiveness of such team treatment would involve experimental units where medical control was suspended, such that leadership could be elected on the basis of skill. Follow-up studies after a 1-year period would be needed to compare the cost and effectiveness of such units with comparable units which had conventional psychiatric leadership. If such studies demonstrated that team leadership were less expensive and more effective than psychiatric leadership, these studies would provide strong incentives for legislative change.

Legal incentive for broad changes in mental health treatment policies are contained in recent court rulings on "right-to-treatment." A recent decision (Wyatt v. Stickney)[6] by the U.S. Fifth Circuit Court contains an extremely detailed listing of the requirements of "Minimum Constitutional Standards for Adequate Treatment of the Mentally Ill." The key item in this list is the requirement of "individualized treatment and posthospital plans" for each patient, which must be developed and implemented within 5 days of admission. The ruling goes on to list the specific contents of the treatment and posthospitalization plans: the problems and needs of the patient, the least restrictive conditions necessary for treatment, long-range and intermediate goals of treatment with a timetable for their attainment, a rationale for these goals and their attainment, a specification of staff responsibility and involvement with the patient, and criteria for release to less restrictive conditions of treatment and for discharge.

In my judgment, there is not a single public mental hospital in the United States that could adequately implement this one aspect of the court order, even if it were applied to new patients only. The manpower (and womanpower) crisis resulting from having to apply it to the backlog of patients already resident further multiplies the magnitude of the problem.

To make implementation of right-to-treatment real, new directions in policy are needed. Policies are needed which could help realize the therapeutic potential of existing treatment staffs and locate new sources of recruitment of therapists: new professions, training for laymen, and possibly ways of utilizing patients as treatment resources for each other. Experiments with team therapy may be an important avenue for exploring new policies in mental health treatment.

SUMMARY

This chapter questions the wisdom of medical dominance of the mental health field. By examining the costs and benefits of the predominant medical treatment, chemotherapy, I have argued that it is not clear that the overall value has been positive. For this reason, it would seem prudent to undertake a program of research that would compare the long-term costs and benefits of team treatment with existing medical practice as a basis for legislative change.

[6]See also Wyatt V. Aderholt (1974).

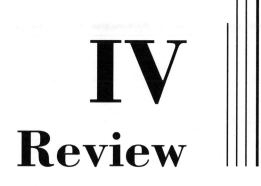

IV
Review

The Labeling Theory
of Mental Illness[1]

12

THE important question one can ask about a theory is whether or not it is true. The next two chapters address the issue of whether or not the labeling theory of mental illness is true. Chapter 12 deals only with my specific theory; Chapter 13 considers the accuracy not only of my labeling approach to mental illness but others as well. At the time of this writing, Walter Gove (1982) still contends that the weight of evidence is very much against the theory. My reading of the current climate of opinion is different, however. In my opinion, sociologists and others are judging that the evidence is mixed: some parts of the theory seem to be supported by the available evidence, others not, and still others not yet tested. Perhaps in the next edition, some parts of the theory can be elaborated, other parts modified or discarded, on the basis of the available evidence.

This chapter presents an evaluation of the labeling theory of mental illness. To this date (1974), there have been three critiques of labeling theory, those by Gove (1970a), Gibbs (1972), and Davis (1972). Gibbs and Davis, for the most part, evaluate formal aspects of the theory; Gove evaluates its substance. Gibbs suggests that the labeling approach is not really a scientific theory in that it is not sufficiently explicit and unambiguous. Davis proposes that there are ideological biases in the labeling approach and points to other approaches as alternatives.[2]

Although the papers by Gibbs and by Davis raise important questions, neither

---

[1] I wish to acknowledge the helpful advice received form Norman Denzin, James Greenley, C. Allen Haney, Arnold Linsky, and William Rushing, who read an earlier draft of this chapter.

[2] For a considered response to the question of bias in labeling theory, see pp. 177–208 in Becker (1973).

considers at length the most fundamental question that can be asked about a theory: How well is it supported by empirical studies? Gove considers this question in his critique, and the present chapter is devoted to it. In the first section of this chapter, I respond to Gove's evaluation, and in the second, I present my own.

First, however, I wish to comment on Gibbs' paper, since it raises a methodological question relevant to assessing evidence presented here. In his analysis of labeling theory, Gibbs demonstrates that the concepts used in the theory are ambiguous, since they are not defined denotatively (i.e., in a way which allows for only a single meaning for each concept). He argues that this ambiguity leaves open many alternative meanings and implications. For this reason, he concludes that the theory in its present state is of little value.

I will make two observations about Gibbs' argument. First, virtually every other sociological theory lacks denotative definition. Indeed, Gibbs observes that the concept of *social norm*, an important element in labeling theory, has never been denotatively defined. Since this concept is perhaps the most basic sociological idea, Gibbs' critique is less an evaluation of labeling theory per se than the state of social science.

Note that Gibbs' critique is equally applicable to psychiatric theories. At this writing, I know of no psychiatric theory of functional mental illness which is based on denotatively defined concepts. The four basic components of the medical model, cause, lesion, symptoms, and outcome, as applied to mental illness are not denotatively defined (this volume, Chapter 14). Nor are such specific concepts as *depression, schizophrenia, phobia,* and *neurosis*. Gibbs' critique of labeling theory, therefore, applies equally well to all of its competitors in the field of mental illness.

My second observation is that Gibbs' critique implies that there is only one kind of science: a positivistic one modeled on natural science. He appears to be saying that a theory has no value unless it can be unambiguously stated. It has been argued, however, that concepts and theories can have a sensitizing function quite distinct from their literal truth value (Blumer, 1954). Theories based on nominal (connotative) definitions can direct attention toward new data or to new ways of perceiving old data, which challenge taken-for-granted assumptions and shatter "the attitude of everyday life" (Bruyn, 1966; Schulz, 1962). In such a view, the very ambiguousness of nominal concepts is of value, since they have a rich evocativeness which denotative concepts lack (Bronowski, 1965).

Science may be viewed as a problem solving activity, with two distinct phases (Bronowski, 1956). In the first phase, the problem is to somehow transcend the traditional classifications and models that imprison thought. In the second, the problem is to test a new idea meticulously. Sensitizing theories are relevant to the first phase of scientific problem solving. They are attempts to jostle the imagination, to create a crisis of consciousness that will lead to new visions of reality. Sensitizing theories are as valuable as denotative theories; they simply attempt to solve a different problem.

The need for new research directions in the study of mental illness has long been apparent. Although thousands of studies have been based on the medical model, real progress toward scientific understanding, or even a fruitful formulation of the problem, is lacking (this volume, Chapter 1: pp. 3–16). The sensitizing function of the labeling theory of mental illness derives precisely from its attempt to contradict the major tenets of the medical model; it is less an attempt to displace that model than to clear the air (see this volume, Chapter 1: pp. 3–16).

It seems to me that none of the three critiques discussed here appreciate the point that a sensitizing theory may be ambiguous, ideologically biased, not literally true, and still be useful and even necessary for scientific progress.

While the labeling theory of mental illness is a sensitizing theory, it can still be used to evaluate evidence in a provisional way. The proper question to ask is not, as Gove asks, whether labeling theory is literally true but whether the relevant studies are more consistent with labeling theory than with its competitor, the medical model. I now turn to this question.

In his critique, Gove reaches the following conclusion: "The available evidence . . . indicates that the societal reaction formulation of how a person becomes mentally ill is substantially incorrect" (1970a: 881). My own reading of the evidence is contrary to that of Gove. First, Gove's interpretation of most studies he cites seems at least questionable and, in some cases, inaccurate. I wish first then to state my objections to several of Gove's interpretations. Second, since Gove's articles were published, several new studies have appeared that have bearing on the controversy. Also, several relevant articles that Gove failed to mention were published earlier than his article. Later in the chapter, I review these articles.

Gove concluded that the majority of the evidence failed to support labeling theory through two kinds of distortion: first, by overstating the implications of those studies he thought refuted labeling theory, and second, by misrepresenting those studies he thought supported labeling theory. I do not try to refute all of Gove's interpretations, since to do so would be to restate labeling theory. I simply indicate some representative errors that he makes.

Apropos of Gove's overstatement, let us examine how he interprets the study by Yarrow *et al.* (1955). To study the processes through which the next-of-kin come to define a person as mentally ill, Yarrow *et al.* interviewed wives of men who had been hospitalized for mental illness. Gove summarizes that study as follows: "Only when the husband's behavior became impossible to deal with would the wife take action to have the husband hospitalized." Gove's interpretation is questionable for two reasons. First, Yarrow *et al.* studied only those cases of deviance that resulted in hospitalization. They did not study all cases of the same type of deviant behavior which led to hospitalization in the entire population. The Yarrow study thus covers only a clinical population and is entirely ex post facto. Gove's interpretation repeats the classic fallacy of the medical model, which is to assume that hospitalization was inevitable even though no observations have been made on the incidence and outcome of similar cases in the unhospitalized population. The history of physical medicine has many analogous cases. For example, it has been found that until the late 1940s, histoplasmosis was thought to be a rare tropical disease with a uniformly fatal outcome (Schwartz and Baum, 1957). Field investigations discovered, however, that the syndrome is widely prevalent and that death or impairment is highly unusual. Analogically, it is possible that the symptoms reported by the wives in Yarrow *et al.* study, even if accurately reported, may terminate without medical intervention.

The question of the accuracy of the wives' report raises the second problem in Gove's interpretation. Yarrow *et al.*'s descriptions of the husbands' behavior are based entirely on the wives' uncorroborated account. Yarrow *et al.* recognize this difficulty, warn the reader about it, and are unassuming about the implications of their findings:

> Ideally to study this problem, one might like to interview the wives as they struggle with the developing illness. This is precluded, however, by the fact that the problem "is not visible" until psychiatric help is sought. The data, therefore, are the wives' reconstructions of their earlier experiences. . . . It is recognized that recollection of the prehospital period may well include systematic biases such as distortions, omissions, and increased organization and clarity [p. 60].

Although Yarrow *et al.* clearly recognize the limitations of their study, Gove does not. He reports the wives' account of the husbands' behavior as if it were the thing itself. Judging from Gove, Laing and Esterson's (1964) detailed study of the way in which the next-of-kin sometimes falsifies his account and colludes against the prepatient may as well have never been written. Laing and Esterson spent an average of 24 hours interviewing members of each of the 11 families in their study, with a range of 16 to 50 hours per family. They found considerable evidence which supported the patient's story rather than the next-of-kin's. For example, in one of their cases, the psychiatrist indicated that the patient, Maya, had "ideas of reference" which supported one of the complaints against her. By interviewing the patient, the mother, and the father together, however, Laing and Esterson put this "delusion" in quite a different light:

> An idea of reference that she had was that something she could not fathom was going on between her parents, seemingly about her. Indeed there was. When they were interviewed together, her mother and father kept exchanging with each other a constant series of nods, winks, gestures, and knowing smiles so obvious to the observer that he commented on them after 20 minutes of the first such interview. They continued, however, unabated and denied [1964:24].

Laing and Esterson found many such items of misrepresentation by the next-of-kin in all their cases. Their study suggests that the uncorroborated account of the next-of-kin is riddled with error.

This is not to say that Laing and Esterson's interpretation is correct and that Gove's is not. I am saying that Yarrow *et al.*'s study and the other studies that Gove cites in this context not only were not organized to test labeling theory, but they were innocent of any of the possible interpretations (such as that of Laing and Esterson) which labeling theory suggests. Until such time as systematic studies are conducted which investigate both clinical and nonclinical populations, and which do not rest entirely on the uncorroborated testimony of one or the other interested parties, interpretations of the kind that Gove makes are dubious.

Another example of how Gove distorts the evidence, seeking to discredit studies which support labeling theory, is his analysis of my article, "The Societal Reaction to Deviance: Ascriptive Elements in the Psychiatric Screening of Mental Patients in a Midwestern State" (Scheff, 1964). The study reported in this article consists of two phases. In the first, preliminary phase, I had hospital psychiatrists rate a sample of incoming patients according to the legal criteria for commitment, dangerousness, and degree of mental impairment. In the second phase, we observed, in a sample of cases, the procedures actually used in committing patients, particularly the psychiatric examination and the formal commitment hearing. The purpose of the psychiatric ratings was to provide a foundation for our observations in the second phase; they were used to determine the extent to which there was any legal uncertainty about the patients' commitability. The second phase of the study described how the judges and psychiatrists reacted to uncertainty. The article stated clearly that the study was divided into two parts: "The purpose of the description that follows is to determine the extent of uncertainty that exists concerning new patients' qualifications for involuntary confinement in a mental hospital, and the reactions of the courts to this type of uncertainty [p. 402]."

In the first phase of the study, the psychiatrists' ratings of the sample of incoming patients were as follows:

Dangerousness

How likely patient would harm self or others (%)		Degree of mental impairment (%)	
Very likely	5	Severe	17
Likely	4	Moderate	42
Somewhat likely	14	Mild	25
Somewhat unlikely	20	Minimal	12
Unlikely	37	None	2
Very unlikely	18		

These findings, it is argued, are relevant to the question of the legal uncertainty concerning the patients' committability. The legal rulings on the presumption of health are stringent. The courts "have repeatedly held that there should be a presumption of sanity. The burden of proof should be on the petitioners (i.e., the next-of-kin). There must be a preponderance of evidence and the evidence should be of a clear and unexceptional nature'' (Scheff, 1964: 403). Given these rulings, it seems reasonable to argue, as the article did, that the committability of all patients except those rated at the extremes of dangerousness or impairment was uncertain. The ratings, it was argued, suggested uncertainty about the committability of 63% of the patients in the sample, (i.e., those patients rated as neither dangerous nor severely impaired).

In the second phase of the study, when we observed the actual commitment procedures, we sought to find out how the psychiatric examiners and judges reacted to uncertainty. To summarize our observations, we found that *all* of the psychiatric examinations and judicial hearings that we witnessed were perfunctory. Furthermore, virtually every hearing resulted in a recommendation for commitment or continued hospitalization. The conclusion of the article is based not on the first phase only but on both phases of the study. Since the first phase suggests uncertainty with respect to the committability of some of the patients, and the second phase suggests that the commitment procedures were perfunctory for the entire sample and yet resulted in continued hospitalization rather than release, in virtually every case, the study appears to demonstrate the presumption of illness.

Gove's treatment of this article is somewhat irresponsible. By ignoring the second phase of the study, he takes the first phase out of context. Ignoring my argument concerning uncertainty, Gove suggests that had I placed the cutting point on the psychiatrists' ratings differently, by including as committable patients rated as moderately impaired and/or somewhat likely to harm themselves, my data "would have shown instead that the vast majority of committed mental patients were mentally ill" (Gove, 1970b). He implies, therefore, that the results of the study rest entirely on my arbitrary choice of a cutting point.[3] In light of all the evidence presented in the article, where the cutting point in the psychiatrists' ratings is placed has little significance. Gove disregarded the problem that the study posed, which was whether or not patients were being committed illegally. He misrepresents my conclusion by imputing to me the conclusion that most of the patients are not mentally ill. The study did not make this point, since I regard the criteria for mental illness as even more ambiguous than the legal standards for commitment.

Gove's other criticism of the study concerns the questionnaire given the psychiatrists, to obtain ratings of dangerousness and mental impairment. He suggests that I should have provided the psychiatrists with descriptions of the behavior that the scales refer to. This criticism begs the question, however, since it seems to assume that there are precise psychiatric or legal criteria of commit-

---

[3]Gove's criticism of the cutting point applies more to an early report of some of the initial results of the study, a brief not in the *American Journal of Psychiatry* (Scheff, 1963). That report acknowledged that setting the cutting point on the psychiatrists' ratings was problematic (p. 268).

table behavior. In fact, the legal statutes, though they vary in language from state to state, are all vague, general, and ambiguous. They state simply that persons who are dangerous or unable to care for themselves may be committed if a strong case can be made. No statutes or psychiatric statements set forth behavioral criteria. My study sought not to help psychiatrists and judges interpret these vague laws but to describe how they reacted to the law's ambiguity.

Some of Gove's criticism seems based on a misunderstanding of labeling theory. He seems to think that showing that the commitment rates reported in various studies are considerably less than 100% somehow refutes labeling theory (Gove, 1970a: 877–879). The argument made by labeling theorists that official agents of the societal reaction usually presume illness does not imply that commitment will always occur any more than presuming innocence in criminal courts implies that acquittal will always occur. The master question which labeling theory raises with respect to commitment rates is more complex than Gove implies. At what point and under what conditions does the process of normalization stop and labeling begin? Gove apparently acknowledges that labeling occurs but only in the last stages of the commitment funnel (i.e., in the formal commitment procedure itself). I suspect that his formulation is much too simple, and that labeling occurs under some conditions much earlier in the process, even in the family or neighborhood; and, conversely, under some conditions, normalization may occur late in the process, as some of my studies showed (this volume, Chapter 5, 6, and 7).

The crucial question we have raised vis-á-vis the medical model concerns contingencies which lead to labeling that lie outside the patient and his behavior. Greenley, for example, established that, independent of a patient's psychiatric condition, the family's desire to bring him home seems to be the most powerful determinant of his length of hospitalization (Greenley, 1972). Labeling theory proposes that the patient's condition is only one of a number of contingencies affecting the societal reaction and, therefore, the patient's fate. Further contingencies are discussed in Chapter 4, (pp. 71, 72), this volume. Gove's interpretation of labeling theory is simplistic and incorrect.

SUMMARIZING THE EVIDENCE

Since most studies of "mental illness" were not designed to test labeling theory, seemingly plausible interpretations of most of them can be constructed either for or against labeling theory. Furthermore, since the conflict between labeling theory and the medical model engenders such furious partisanship, we should also exclude studies based on casual or unsystematic observations in which the observers' bias are more likely to influence the results he reports. I have surveyed the research literature, therefore, for studies that meet two criteria. First, they must relate to labeling theory explicitly; and, second, the research methods must be systematic. At this writing, I have located 18 studies of this type. Of these eighteen only 5, those by Gove (1973, 1974), Karmel

(1969, 1970) and Robbins (1966) are inconsistent with labeling theory; the remainder, those of Denzin (1968), Denzin and Spitzer (1966), Greenley (1972), Haney and Michielutte (1968), Haney, Miller and Michielutte (1969), Linsky (1970a, b), Rosenhan (1973), Rushing (1971), Scheff (1964), Temerlin (1968), Wilde (1968), and Wenger and Fletcher (1969) are consistent with labeling theory.

These 18 studies vary widely in the reliability of the inferences that we can make from them. Four studies among those consistent with labeling theory use zero-order correlations—those of Denzin and Spitzer (1966); Denzin (1968); Haney and Michielutte (1968); and Haney, Miller, and Michielutte (1969). For example, Haney reports the correlation between the decision to commit and social characteristics of the patients and petitioners. He finds positive correlations between commitment rates and these social characteristics. For example, he reports a higher rate of commitment for nonwhites than whites. Although his findings are consistent with labeling theory, they provide only very weak support, since he has not controlled for the patient's condition. We are left with the question that occurs so often in social epidemiology: Are nonwhites committed more often because of the societal reaction to their social status or because this particular social status is itself correlated with mental illness? That is to say, are nonwhites committed more often than whites because of their powerlessness or because there is more mental illness among them? Haney's studies do not answer such questions, nor do those of Denzin and Spitzer (1966), and Denzin (1968).

Similar criticism can be made of the two studies by Karmel (1969, 1970) which fail to support labeling theory. Based on interviews with patients after their hospitalization, her data fail to show any evidence of the acceptance of a deviant role predicted by labeling theory. These are simple correlation studies with no controls (Bohr, 1970). Gove (1973) studied the amount and effects of stigma on a sample of ex-mental patients. His data indicate that the amount and effects of stigma were not very large and therefore fail to support labeling theory. His data are somewhat ambiguous, however, since there is no control group of similar persons who were not hospitalized.

A series of much stronger studies whose findings support labeling theory are those of Greenley (1972), Rushing (1972), Linsky (1972), Scheff (1964), Wenger and Fletcher (1969), and Wilde (1968). My study has already been discussed. Greenley (1972), as indicated, studied the relationship between length of hospitalization and several social and psychiatric variables. He found that even when the patient's psychiatric condition is controlled, there is a strong relationship between the family desire for the patient's release and the length of hospitalization.

Rushing and Linsky each did studies on the relationship between psychiatric commitment and social class and other social characteristics. Since they indicated that their data only partly overlap, I will cite both studies (Linsky, 1972; Rushing, 1972). Both used the same technique, which I believe controls for the patient's condition. If they had merely used commitment rates as their dependent variable, we would be left with the perplexing question: are commitment rates higher in the lowest social class because there is more mental illness in that class or for other reasons? (See the New Haven studies by Hollinghead and Redlich [1958].) However, both Rushing and Linsky used an index made up of the ratio of involuntary to voluntary hospital admissions, as a measure of societal reaction. I believe that such a ratio will control for gross variations in rates of mental illness. What the index provides, hopefully, is a measure of the most severe societal reaction (i.e., involuntary confinement) but with the phenomenon of mental illness at least partly controlled, assuming that the voluntary comitments are equally "mentally ill." Perhaps this assumption should also be investigated. Both studies show a strong relationship between powerlessness and commitment rates. In the study by Wenger and Fletcher (1969), the presence of a lawyer representing the patient in admission hearings decreased the likelihood of hospitalization. This relationship held within three degrees of manifest "mental illness."

Finally, Wilde's study (1968) concerns the relationship between the recommendations for commitment made by mental health examiners and various social characteristics of the prepatients, with controls for the patient's psychiatric condition. In all five of these studies strong relationships are reported between such social characteristics as class and commitment rates, with psychiatric conditions controlled for. These five studies support labeling theory since they indicate that social characteristics of the patients help determine the severity of the societal reaction, independent of psychiatric condition.

The controlled studies by Robbins (1966) and by Gove (1974) provide data that fail to support labeling theory. Robbins used psychiatric diagnoses of adults who had been diagnosed as children as part of an evaluation of child guidance clinics. Robbins noted that some of the children diagnosed were treated and some were not. She argues that this data can be used to evaluate the effects of "the severity of societal response to the behavior problems of the children." She found that of the adults who had psychiatric treatment as children, 16% were diagnosed as having sociopathic personalities as adults. Of the persons who did not receive psychiatric treatment as children, 24% were diagnosed as having sociopathic personalities as adults. Since the difference between the two percentages is not statistically significant, the hypothesis that psychiatric treatment was beneficial is not supported, but by the same token, neither is the labeling hypothesis that psychiatric treatment, particularly when involuntary, may stabilize behavior that would otherwise be transient. This finding is somewhat equivocal, however, because of the sampling problems of the original Cambridge–Somerville study.

With a sample of hospitalized mental patients, Gove (1974) has studied the relationship between the patient's psychiatric record and his economic and social resources. His data suggest that individual resources facilitate treatment rather than allow the individual to avoid the societal reaction and, therefore, support the medical model rather than labeling theory. Some caution is necessary in interpreting these findings, however, since patient characteristics were based on hospital data. For example, he finds that more of the records of patients with low resources present the patient as "never psychiatrically normal" than patients with higher resources. Does this mean that low resource patients have been "mentally ill" longer, or that the hospital tends to construct their case histories in this way, retroactively (Goffman, 1961:145)? In any case, Gove's interpretation of his data contradicts the conclusions of Linsky (1972) and of Rushing (1972). Since the studies do not use the same indices, it is not possible to compare them directly.

The final two studies to be discussed provide still stronger support for labeling theory. The first, Temerlin's (1968), is a test of the influence of suggestion on psychiatric diagnosis. Temerlin finds that psychiatrists and clinical psychologists are extremely suggestible when it comes to diagnosing mental illness. Four different groups diagnosed the patient in the same recorded interview under different conditions. One control group diagnosed with no prior suggestion, one group was given a suggestion that the interviewee was sane, and a third group was told that they were selecting scientists to work in research. In the experimental group, it was suggested that the interviewees were mentally ill. The diagnoses of the control and experimental groups differed greatly. In the control groups, the great majority made diagnoses of mental health; whereas in the experimental group, not a single psychiatrist out of 25 and only 3 out of 25 psychologists diagnosed mental health. One weakness of this study is that it takes place in an artificial setting with an enacted interview; but it strongly supports the unreliability of psychiatric diagnosis and the presumption of illness.

The study by Rosenhan (1973) took place in real settings—12 mental hospitals. For this study, eight sane persons gained secret admittance to the different hospitals. They all followed the same plan. In his initial admission interview, each pseudopatient simulated several psychotic symptoms. Immediately upon admission to the ward, the pseudopatients stopped simulating the symptoms of abnormality. In all 12 cases, the pseudopatients had enormous difficulty establishing that they were sane. The length of hospitalization ranged from 7 to 52 days with an average of 19 days. The study's major finding is as follows:

> Despite their public show of sanity, the pseudo-patients were never detected. Admitted except in one case with a diagnosis of schizophrenia, each was discharged with a diagnosis of schizophrenia in remission. The label "in remission" should in no way be dismissed as a formality for at no time during any hospitalization had any question been raised about any pseudo-patient's simulation . . . the evidence is strong that once labeled schizophrenic the pseudo-patient was stuck with the label [p. 252].

Rosenhan also collected a wide variety of subsidiary data dealing with the amount and quality of contact between the pseudopatients and the hospital staff, showing a strong tendency for the staff to treat the pseudopatients as nonpersons.

This study, like Temerlin's (1968), strongly supports labeling theory. Both provide good models for future studies of labeling theory: the Rosenhan study with its use of actual hospital locations and the Temerlin study with its experimental design.

We can now provisionally summarize the state of evidence concerning labeling theory. If we restrict ourselves to systematic studies explicitly related to labeling theory, 18 are available. Of these 13 support labeling theory and 5 fail to. Although the studies vary in reliability and precision the balance of evidence seems to support labeling theory.

The Labeling
Theory Paradigm

13

In this chapter, I comment on several aspects of labeling theory. First, I discuss the state of the art with respect to evidence: At this time (1979), to what extent is the theory supported by empirical evidence? This discussion begins with an assessment of the controversy over the Rosenhan (1973) study, since this study has stirred the most interest of all the current labeling studies. The discussion of evidence continues with my commentary on an article by Krohn and Akers (1979), which assesses the relevance of studies of the hospitalization and discharge of mental patients to the dispute over the validity of psychiatric and labeling models. Next, I discuss a recent study of hospitalization decisions by Feigelson and his collaborators (1978) in terms of its implications for labeling theory. Finally, in the conclusion I outline two new directors in the study of labeling: first, the development of positive and negative labels and valuations, and second, the study of the collective psychodynamic sources of labeling.

The labeling theory of mental illness is founded on the idea that what are called "symptoms of mental illness" can also be conceptualized as a certain kind of nonconformity: the violation of residual rules. Every society has myriad explicit rules and understandings about appropriate behavior, perceptions, feelings, and thoughts. For every explicit rule (e.g., stay on the right side of the road), however, there are probably many more rules that are so taken for granted that they are never stated or even thought about. It goes without saying, for example, that in conversation one may look at the eyes and mouth of the speaker but not gaze only at his/her ear. When a person's behavior is disruptive or upsetting and we cannot find a conventional label of deviance (crime, drunkenness, etc.), we may resort to a miscellaneous or residual category. In earlier societies, witchcraft or spirit or demonic possession were used. In our society, our residual category is mental illness.

This is not to claim, of course, that some symptoms of mental illness are not caused by disease. For example, it is clear that some hallucinations and delusions have their origins in illness, as in the case of general paresis. But it is also true that the violation of residual rules may be generated by other causes: stress, such as sleep deprivation; psychological causes, such as conditioning, and finally, volitional acts of innovation or defiance, as in artistic creation or religious movements. Residual rule-breaking may have its origins in complex combinations of two or more of these sources: organic causes, environmental stress, psychological causes, or volition.

Since there appears to be a virtually infinite number of causes, the strategy of the labeling approach is to avoid the question of the causation of the original deviance and to concentrate on a question that is usually ignored: Given residual rule-breaking, from whatever cause, why are some short-lived or self-limited and others stable? The hypothesis offered by the theory concerns the societal reaction to residual rule-breaking: Residual rule-breaking, which is normalized by the rule-breaker and/or others, will usually not stabilize. Conversely, rule-breaking that is labeled (i.e., stigmatized and segregated) may lead to a career of deviance.

As already indicated in Chapters 3 and 4, the theory can be stated as a set of nine propositions:

1. Residual rule-breaking arises from fundamentally diverse sources.
2. Relative to the rate of treated mental illness, the rate of unrecorded residual rule-breaking is extremely high.
3. Most residual rule-breaking is normalized and is of transitory significance.
4. Stereotyped imagery of mental disorder is learned in early childhood.
5. The stereotypes of insanity are continually reaffirmed, inadvertently, in ordinary social interaction.
6. Labeled deviants may be rewarded for playing the stereotyped deviant role.
7. Labeled deviants are punished when they attempt the return to conventional roles.
8. In the crisis occurring when a residual rule-breaker is publicly labeled, the deviant is highly suggestible and may accept the proffered role of the insane as the only alternative.
9. Among residual rule-breakers, labeling is the single most important cause of careers of residual deviance.[1]

---

[1]The *contingencies* that govern the severity of the societal reaction and therefore whether labeling or normalization will occur, may be considered as part of Proposition 9.

For a review of the 7 contingencies that lead to labeling and the societal reaction see this volume, Chapter 4 (pp. 71, 72).

The contingencies that have figured most prominently in published research have been the degree of deviance and the power of the rule-breaker. The other five contingencies have received relatively little attention.

The purpose of labeling theory is not to replace psychiatric or psychological approaches but to complement them by emphasizing that ''mental illness'' may be at least as much a social fact as it is a physical fact. By emphasizing, even exaggerating, the social and reflexive character of much of human behavior, labeling theory may serve as a corrective to the misuse of the medical model of mental illness and point to a synthesis of individual and collective models.

THE ROSENHAN STUDY

The labeling study that has recently received the most attention in the scientific world was conducted by a Stanford psychologist, David Rosenhan. He arranged to have 8 persons, himself and 7 confederates, seek admission in 12 different hospitals, each person feigning a single psychiatric symptom: hearing voices. If admitted, each person was to immediately drop all feigning. The object of the study was to see if normal persons would be admitted under these circumstances, and if admitted, how long it would take for them to be released, and how they would be treated until release.

To repeat the outcome: admission occurred in all 12 cases; the diagnosis of schizophrenia was made in 11 cases and manic-depressive psychosis in one case. The mean time until release was 19 days, with a range of from 7 to 52 days. All were discharged with the diagnosis ''schizophrenia in remission.'' In addition to these findings, the study reported data on attempts to converse with hospital personnel, showing that the patients were treated like nonpersons.

The study was published in *Science* (1973), where it created, by the norms of that journal, a storm of protest. There were 15 letters published in the issue of April 27. Many of the letter writers appeared to be psychiatrists. In 1975, there was also a substantial response from psychologists in a symposium in the *Journal of Abnormal Psychology,* which contained five articles, all of which were strongly critical. These articles, and the letters in *Science* as well, raise a whole host of conceptual and methodological questions about the study and one ethical question.

Several of the commentators criticized the ethics of the study, since it involved deception of the staffs of the hospitals studies. A second ethical question which was not raised by the critics, but might well have been, concerns the risks to the pseudopatients themselves. Aside from risks incurred during the average stay of 19 days, there would appear to be risks which might have continued after release. It is conceivable that an episode of admission to a mental hospital appearing in their records could be an embarrassment to the participants at some point in their later lives. Rosenhan's finding that all the psuedopatients were released with the diagnosis "in remission" rather than "cured" supports the idea that there may be something indelible about psychiatric treatment. The fate of Senator Eagleton, the initial nominee for Vice President in the McGovern campaign, illustrates this phenomenon.

In my judgment, any study involving either of these ethical issues, deception of staff or risks to participants, represents a very high cost. The possible benefits of Rosenhan's study, since it involves both costs, would have to be very great indeed to outweigh these costs. Do the benefits of the study outweigh the costs? In the framework within which Rosenhan presents the study, as a test of diagnostic accuracy, I would have to concur with his critics. The results are neither clear nor conclusive tests of diagnostic accuracy. If this were the case, the study probably should not have been done. However, in the discussion below, I suggest how the framework may be revised, so that, with some additional research, the results of the study may yield a sufficiently high benefit to outweigh the costs. First, however, I describe some of the other points made by Rosenhan's critics.

All of the critics agree that the conclusion that Rosenhan drew from his data, that "psychiatric hospitals . . . cannot distinguish the sane from the insane," was much too broad. The inference that the critics suggest as correct may be something like: the hospitals in the study could not distinguish persons who were feigning psychiatric symptoms from persons who were not feigning. Several critics point out that a similar result may occur in some areas in general medicine: people with "Munchausen syndrome" (i.e., those who fake illness so well that they receive treatment) or people feigning the symptoms of heart disease, low back pain, or headache.

Most of the criticism concerned the design of the research as well as the inferences that were drawn from the findings. Virtually all of the critics point out that the absence of controls make interpretation of the findings difficult. For example, one of the critics, Millon (1975), suggests the need for blind controls: confederates who are unaware of the hypothesis of the study. He proposes that because of the demand characteristics of the experimentor's expectation, the confederates might not have tried to be released so much as they would have if they were not aware of the hypothesis. Millon, as well as several other critics, propose a number of alternate designs: a condition in which normal persons try to get admitted without any feigning of symptoms; a condition in which real patients from one hospital would seek admission at another hospital with no feigning; and finally, a group of diagnosticians could be asked to discriminate among a group composed equally of real patients and pseudopatients.

Rosenhan's focus on the accuracy of psychiatric diagnosis in an absolute sense (can hospitals tell the sane from the insane?) allows Farber (1975), in his lengthy article, to rehearse the entire history of psychodiagnosis in all of its conceptual, methodological, and even philosophical complexity. Farber (1975: p. 589) criticizes Rosenhan's paper as a "melange of epistomological assumptions, theoretical inferences, and empirical data, the complete unscrambling of which requires greater conversance than I have with highly technical issues in philosophy of science, taxonomic logic, theories of psychopathology, and psychodiagnostic theory and practice.'' Farber refers Rosenhan to a standard work on psychodiagnosis (Meehl, 1973), suggesting that in that work, basic issues that Rosenhan does not even consider are treated in a consistent and lucid manner.

I now present my own position by responding first to Rosenhan's critics and then to the original study itself. I find my self in agreement with many of the critic's points about the study's concepts and methods. I agree with Farber's point about the many ways in which the study is inadequate to the task of testing the hypothesis. I find it ironic that Rosenhan phrases the hypothesis of the study in terms of the legal–medical concepts of sanity and insanity. The study and its results represent a protest against the use of these concepts. The attack is confounded, however, because it utilizes the very ideas that it is attacking. As indicated previously, it is possible to construct a sociological model of the societal reaction, that allows the researcher to formulate problems and hypotheses concerning "mental illness" in a language that does not depend on the assumptions of the medical–legal model (see Chapter 13, this volume).

However, I believe that there is another framework that will salvage Rosenhan's results, which speaks directly to the conflict between Rosenhan and his critics. As already indicated, many of the critics allude to comparisons between psychodiagnosis and diagnosis in physical medicine. Farber (1975: p. 589) comes closest to making this comparison explicit, in one of his conclusions: "The reliability of psychodiagnostic classification . . . is not demonstrably poorer than many useful diagnostic groupings in general medicine." I believe that the comparison between psychiatry and physical medicine lies at the heart of the controversy, although I would not phrase the comparison in the way that Farber has. First of all, I think that Farber does not mean what he says: He refers to the *reliability* (i.e., repeatability) of psychiatric diagnosis when he means *validity* (i.e., accuracy). Second, the criteria he mentions, usefullness, seems to me somewhat ambiguous and vague; useful to whom, in what specific ways? Finally, and most important, I find fault with the main thrust of his conclusion: that psychiatric diagnosis is "not demonstrably poorer" than diagnosis in general medicine. I know of no demonstrations either pro or con of this point. It is to this issue, I think, that the focus of the study should be shifted.

Why is the comparison between psychiatry and the rest of medicine so important? It is important, I think, because the belief that psychiatry is not unlike general medicine is a metahypothesis, a belief so primitive that it goes unstated, and therefore untested, in most research, discussion, and, most powerfully, in most legislation concerning mental disorder. The mental health ethos of our times was launched by an advertising campaign by the National Association for Mental Health, based on the slogan "Mental illness is an illness just like any other." The intent of this campaign was to remove the aura of stigma and hopelessness that surrounded popular conceptions of mental disorder. The campaign helped convert the public image of mental disorder to the medical model and, therefore, perhaps, raised the status of mental disorder. At the same time, however, public acceptance of the medical model crystallized psychiatric dominance of the field by legislative fiat. By law as well as custom, mental disorder is owned by psychiatric medicine. Of all the aspects of the vast and chaotic field of mental disorder, medical hegemony may be the most irrational, since the fiscal and intellectual problems it creates are self-inflicted.

Psychiatric dominance rests on the untested assumption that psychiatric treatment is basically similar to other medical treatments. Rosenhan's study could be used to challenge that assumption. The point that the psychologist Neisser (1973) makes in the sole favorable letter to *Science* is relevant:

> psychiatric diagnoses, unlike those in other branches of medicine, are almost irreversible. Internists, neurologists, and pediatricians sometimes have to admit errors, but a psychiatrist never does; it is not he who was remiss, but the schizophrenia which is in remission . . .
> A medical diagnosis is much like a hypothesis in science; it should lead to further predictions and be subject to disconfirmation. In science, hypotheses that cannot be disproved by any conceivable evidence are not hypotheses at all. Should we not conclude that diagnoses which cannot be disproved are equally meaningless? By showing that the diagnosis of "schizophrenia" is essentially irreversible, no matter how the patient subsequently behaves, Rosenhan has dealt the scientific pretensions of psychiatry a serious blow.

Neisser's explicit comparison of psychiatry with the rest of medicine is helpful as is his discussion of the similiarity between a diagnosis and a hypothesis. However, he and Farber make a similar error, but in opposite directions: Farber assumes, without test, that the level of psychiatric misdiagnosis is comparable with general medicine; Neisser assumes, without test, that in general medicine, diagnoses are more reversible than they are in psychiatry. The question would appear to require empirical testing: (*a*) the hypothesis of the study becomes comparative rather than absolute; (*b*) the level of error in psychiatry is significantly higher than in general medicine; (*c*) pseudopatients feigning a symptom of a physical illness would be admitted to general hospitals at a lower rate than in Rosenhan's study, the mean detention time would be significantly shorter than 19 days, and, in those cases where the hospital was fooled, the reversal of the initial diagnosis would occur more frequently than zero.

To be sure, the completion of Rosenhan's design in this way, by adding a comparison of the reaction to feigned illness in general medicine, does not involve a complete test of the hypothesis that the practice of psychiatry is significantly different from the practice of the rest of medicine. As some of the critics pointed out, success in detecting feigning may not be the most important criterion that one could use in evaluating a profession. For example, the cure rate, expense, length of treatment, and absence of side effects of treatment are more crucial criteria, from a practical point of view. A comprehensive test of the hypothesis would require comparisons of psychiatry and general medicine along these dimensions as well as ability to detect feigning. Furthermore, a comprehensive test would also require comparison along these various criteria with respect to the major syndromes that are usually treated, rather than just a single syndrome, as was done by Rosenhan.

Nevertheless, the Rosenhan study is a beginning step in the right direction. His results can be interpreted as sampling one important aspect that a comprehensive comparison between medicine and psychiatry would survey. The results of larger scale study, which would make explicit comparisons with several syndromes along several dimensions, would surely be valuable for both scientific and public policy purposes. To the extent that the hypothesis is supported, it may be possible to accelerate the sharing of power between psychiatry and the other mental health professions and to clarify some of the conceptual and methodological problems brought about by the excessive emphasis on the medical model of mental disorder.

Also pointing in this direction is an extremely important series of studies conducted by Aaron Lazare and his associates (1975a, 1975b). Lazare trained his psychiatric co-workers to notice and respond to requests that psychiatric patients make. His studies suggest that typically in psychiatric interviews, the therapist is so intent on making a diagnosis that he ignores implicit or even explicit requests patients may make. He has developed a list of requests that patients may endorse: clarification, expertise, insight, control, ventilation, medication, succorance, reality contact, advice, community triage (as in locating social agencies relevant to patient's problems), confession, and so on. In Lazare's method, the therapist does not necessarily accede to the patient's request, but he at least acknowledges it. If the therapist does not wish to give the patient what he/she wants, the therapist will offer some alternatives. This technique transforms the patient from a passive to an active agent in the interaction by leading to negotiation over treatment. It also changes the major function of the therapist from being a diagnostic labeler to a negotiator, a skill which can be learned more cheaply in many settings other than in medical school. The broadening of the occupational base for therapists to give full membership to clinical psychology, social work, and other professions is a necessary next step in this field.

The next issue concerns the scientific status of labeling theory. In 1976, I published a report which evaluated the evidence for and against the theory (see Chapter 12, this volume). I noted at that time that the evaluation must be provisional, since most of the relevant studies were not designed to compare labeling theory with the medical model of mental illness. I reported 18 studies whose results seemed relevant to the controversy; 13 supported labeling theory, 5 did not. Keeping in mind the provisional nature of the evaluation, I concluded that the balance of evidence at that time favored labeling theory.

Recently, a similar assessment has been made using more refined categories and a larger group of studies. Krohn and Akers (1977) assessed the results of 26 studies concerning the determinants of admission and discharge of mental patients. Their conclusions are similar to mine. They find that 23 of the studies support labeling theory, and only three do not (see their chart, p. 346). Furthermore, they are quite critical of two of the three studies that fail to support labeling theory. They point out that both of these studies, which were conducted by Gove and his collaborators, involved an unusual hospital which was experimenting with a short-term, intensive care demonstration treatment program. They conclude that the program was quite atypical of mental hospitals. For example, members of patients' families were included in 83% of all counseling sessions, and weekend visits home were encouraged. The majority of the patients were admitted voluntarily.

Krohn and Akers (1977: 343) go on to make an important point about the relevance of the involuntary–voluntary distinction to tests of labeling theory not only in connection with the Gove studies but for all studies of admission and discharge:

> Gove and Howell (1974) interpret their finding that people with more social resources (i.e., higher income and married) are more likely to be admitted to the mental hospital as contradicting the societal reaction model. They dismiss the voluntary–involuntary distinction as either unimportant (to the psychiatric perspective) or unclear (in the labeling perspective). And yet, it is the very fact that two-thirds of their sample were voluntary admissions which casts doubt on their interpretation. Labeling proponents have emphasized relative power in the process by which unwanted labels are imposed on individuals; they have not been much concerned with label seeking. Thus the perspective's insights are most applicable to questions about resisting the imposition or maintenance of labels. . . . However, to the extent that power is also important in attaining positively desired goals, one could hypothesize, consistent with labeling, that there is a positive relationship between social resources and hospitalization among voluntary patients—precisely what Gove and Howell found.

Krohn and Akers are critical not only of the studies that fail to support labeling theory but also of the studies that do support it. They indicate that of the 26 studies they reviewed, half had no controls. That is, 13 of the studies did not control either for psychiatric variables or for social variables. Looked at the other way, however, of the 13 studies which did include controls, only one study failed to support labeling theory, and this one study, by Gove and Fain (1975), is one of those suggested by Krohn and Akers to be only partially relevant to labeling theory because it was conducted in a highly atypical hospital. As in Chapter 12, Krohn and Akers (1977: 341) conclude with provisional support for labeling theory: "The research does not allow for unequivocal conclusions, but there is a clear tendency for admission and discharge of mental patients to be related more to social than to psychiatric variables, particularly when the patients are unwilling to be committed or retained."

They end their paper with the suggestion that social learning theory may provide an alternative to both the labeling and psychiatric view of the determinants of the decisions which affect mental patients. They argue that mental health personnel may act either as control agents for society or as therapeutic agents acting on behalf of their patients, and that this outcome may be determined by the reinforcement schedule for the personnel. I am in complete agreement with this argument. In several of my own studies, I have described the social sanctions which influence legal psychiatric decisions. I would disagree, however, that social learning theory is an alternative to labeling theory. I would see it, rather, as complementary. Labeling theory is one aspect of a broader theory of social control, in which social norms are upheld by sanctions: positive sanctions for conformity, negative sanctions for nonconformity. Although the terminology is different (in learning theory, punishment and reward would be substituted for negative and positive sanctions), the idea is basically the same. Another difference is that the focus in labeling theory has been on the social control of the rule-breakers rather than of the rule-enforcers, as suggested by Krohn and Akers. Their suggestion should be interpreted as the inclusion of the rule-enforcers as an additional part of the total system of social control rather than as an alternative theoretical perspective.

Although the review by Krohn and Akers has been helpful for evaluating the status of labeling theory, the evaluation is quite provisional. Their review covered only a small group of studies that are relevant: studies of admission and discharge. A complete review of the evidence would need to cover many other areas of the literature. Three areas are cited as examples: longitudinal studies, experiments on labeling and suggestion, and studies of the effects of treatment. To begin with the topic of longitudinal studies: In an earlier paper with Sundstrom (this volume, Chapter 9), I reassessed a review by Clarizio (1968) of studies of the stability of deviant behavior over time. Our reassessment supported the labeling theory hypothesis that most symptomatic behavior, particularly in childhood, seems to be transitory. However, this issue probably should be reopened. Our review was at one remove, since we reinterpreted studies gathered by another researcher. Also, since 10 years have passed since the original review, additional studies are probably now available.

A second set of studies which requires review and critical assessment are experiments on the effects of labeling or suggestion on diagnosis, such as those by Temerlin (1968), Caetano (1974), and Lebedun and Collins (1976). These studies show that psychodiagnosticians are strongly influenced by suggestion in making diagnoses on the basis of hearing a taped interview or seeing the film of an interview. For example, in the Temerlin study, a prestigeful confederate of the researcher's, a well-known senior psychologist, remarked before the subjects heard a sound-recorded interview, "the patient is a very interesting man because he looks neurotic, but actually is quite psychotic." After hearing this suggestion, the majority of psychiatrists who served as subjects diagnosed the patient as psychotic. In the control condition, with no suggestion, none of the psychiatrists diagnosed psychosis. If we accept the results as valid, they support the labeling theory hypothesis that labeling, rather than normalization, may be a result of contingencies in addition to psychopathological symptoms.

One question that has been raised about these results is whether one may generalize from an experiment using a standard stimulus to an actual diagnostic situation. A second question concerns the informational status of the suggestion. Farber (1975), in his comments on the Rosenhan study, has suggested that the presence of a person seeking admission to a mental hospital carries valuable information to a diagnostician. Even though in a particular case it may be misleading, as it was with the pseudopatients, nevertheless, he says, it has predictive value in that most people who seek admission will have real symptoms. A similar comment may also be made about the studies such as those by Temerlin (1968); even though the suggestion made by a fellow diagnostician was misleading in this particular context, in most cases, it will have actuarial value for prediction. My own reaction to this argument is to try to transform it into a researchable question. As in the case of the Rosenhan study, I would suggest that the issue of the informational value of suggestions be put in the context of a comparison with physical medicine. If physicians were diagnosing a physical illness on the basis of exposure to comparable evidence, say an X-ray film, would a comparable suggestion have as much effect on their diagnoses? My guess would be that it would not: In physical medicine, diagnosticians would be little influenced by suggestion unless it was accompanied by additional evidence (which was not the case in studies at issue). This and other methodological issues connected with the experiments probably require additional evaluation and commentary, however.

Finally, studies of the effects of treatment on mental illness probably should be reviewed for their relevance to labeling theory. This is a much larger literature than those discussed earlier. However, a systematic review and evaluation may provide another source for the provisional testing of labeling hypotheses. One may be able to make a rough distinction between treatments which involved segregation and/or stigmatization as against those that did not. If one could assume matched populations, the hypothesis to be evaluated would be that to the extent a treatment avoided stigmatization and/or segregation (as in containment strategies in military psychiatry); to that extent, it would result in less chronicity than those treatments that did not. Evidence of this kind, together with reviews of longitudinal studies and experiments, would provide a more extended basis for evaluation of labeling theory than the one that is offered here.

To complete this review of the current status of labeling theory, I would like to refer to a new study which has appeared since the publication of the Krohn and Akers article. This study, "The Decision to Hospitalize" by Feigelson et al. (1978), appeared in the *American Journal of Psychiatry*. It is of more than ordinary interest for several reasons. First, it is a study of the determinants of hospitalization conducted by a group of psychiatrists, it appeared in the leading psychiatric journal and suggested that the kinds of issues with which labeling theory has been concerned are increasing in importance in psychiatry. Second, unlike many of the earlier studies of admission, the study allows for the direct comparison of the importance of psychiatric and social determinants of hospitalization, since it employs multiple regression analysis. Finally, the article is marked by a number of errors that I would like to correct.

The study was conducted because the authors noted that in the psychiatric services of four New York City hospitals in 1974, the hospitalization rates varied from a low of 16% in one hospital to a high 57% in another. The question which the study seemed to address was: do the variations in hospitalization rates merely reflect variations in the severity of illness of the incoming patients, or do they reflect variations in the screening practices of the hospitals? To answer this question, the authors took a sample of 50 patients seen in the emergency service of each of the hospitals. The patients in ths sample were interviewed by psychiatrists on the staff of the research project and were rated as to severity of symptoms on a Global Assessment Scale and also rated as to whether or not they were psychotic, chronic, and had been previously hospitalized. The results are reported in Table 13.1.

TABLE 13.1   Stagewise Multiple Regression Analysis of Determinants of Psychiatric Hospitalization[a]

Independent variable	r^2	r^2 Change	Significance
Global assessment score	.05477	.05477	p 0.01
Psychotic illness	.05478	.00001	n.s.[b]
Chronic illness	.05712	.00235	n.s.[b]
Previous hospitalization	.09075	.03363	p 0.05
Hospitals (df = 3)	.18450	.09375	p 0.01

[a]From Feigelson *et al.* (1978:356).
[b]Data not significant.

The authors interpret these results as showing that the "nature and severity of a patient's problems played the most important role in the decision to hospitalize . . . " This is a curious reading of the table, since it is clear that the hospital variable accounts for the largest proportion of the variance (9.375%). They argue that the other variables, which they interpret as reflecting the nature and severity of the patient's problems, are more important since they appeared first in the regression equation. However, it seems likely that the order in which the variables appeared is an artifact of the types of variables used in the study and of the particular multiple regression method used. In the method they used, stagewise multiple regression, the variables appear in the equation according to the size of their zero-order correlation with the dependent variable. Since they used four highly intercorrelated psychiatric variables and only one nonpsychiatric variable, the zero-order coefficients are speciously large. A correct reading of their findings would be that what Krohn and Akers call an extrapsychiatric variable, the hospital variable, accounts for the largest proportion of the variance in the decision to hospitalize; indeed, more than all of the psychiatric variables combined.

The selection of the variables in the study is important for another reason. The authors interpret their findings to show that "the decision to hospitalize was firmly based on the nature and severity of a patient's problems . . ." The use of the word firmly in this conclusion is ironic, since all of the psychiatric variables combined account for less than 10% of the variance, leaving more than 90% unaccounted for. Even if one includes the hospital variable, more than 80% of the variance is still unaccounted for. The major finding of the study, it seems to me, is that the authors are unable to account for most of the variance in the decision to hospitalize and have, therefore, been unable to demonstrate that they understand its causes.

Perhaps if the authors had included variables in addition to the five that they used, they could have explained the hospitalization decision more effectively. This issue suggests a final criticism of the study. In the Krohn and Akers review, 20 studies of the determinants of admission are listed. Feigelson *et al.* (1978) do not cite a single one of these studies, even though they are all concerned with exactly the same topic that they studied. Nor is there any citation of the considerable literature on labeling theory. Either of these sources would have offered many suggestions for social variables additional to the ones they studied. I would suggest that the time has come when studies of psychiatric decisions should involve diverse social variables as well as the usual psychiatric ones.

NEW DIRECTIONS

My assessment of the current status of labeling studies leads me to several conclusions. First, existing studies have established that labeling theory is at least as powerful as the more conventional psychiatric approaches that are usually used in the study of psychiatric decision making. It would follow that future studies should routinely include labeling concepts and hypotheses as part of there approach. Fifteen years ago, it seemed important to me that both psychiatric and labeling hypotheses should be tested in the same study to compare their effectiveness. Today, such a comparison seems to be less important. What seems important now is that both perspectives be used in order to increase the power of the analysis. The scope and complexity of the issues involved in the study of mental disorder suggest the need for an interdisciplinary approach.

In the brief space that follows, I suggest two areas for future research which would require interdisciplinary cooperation. The first area concerns long-term changes in the societal reaction in a historical perspective. It seems to me that progress in the development of labeling theory may be faster if it were applied to problems broader than contemporary issues of mental illness. For example, it may be of great significance to trace the development of tests for the authenticity of religious visions that occurred in the Catholic church in the Middle Ages. The concept of *hallucination* as a symptom is a relatively modern invention, since in most of human history, visions have been usually accepted as parts of reality rather than as manifestations of deviance.

Labeling theory could also be applied to areas other than mental disorder. Two important questions come to mind. The first concerns the development of justifications for taking human life: the distinction between killing and murder. The sources for changes in the societal reaction to killing are surely worth knowing, since they could increase our understanding of genocide and the development of the modern institution of total war. A similar type of study would be to trace the sources of changes in the societal reaction to the kind of behavior that may be referred to as ''hoarding'' in a society based on sharing but in modern industrial societies would be given a positive label, such as ''capital accumulation.'' I believe that labeling theorists have been excessively preoccupied with problems that have been defined by other professions (e.g., psychiatry) as important and have not sufficiently defined problems for themselves.

The last suggestion I wish to make for interdisciplinary collaboration concerns the problem of the sources of labeling, which may require cooperation between sociologists and clinical psychologists. It seems to me that in order to explain the virtually universal phenomena of the labeling, segregation, and stigmatization of deviants, it may be necessary to study the collective psychodynamics of the feelings that members of the society have about its deviants. Stigmatization rests primarily upon strong emotions of fear, angers and embarrassment. Much of this emotional charge seems to be vicarious, in that persons who have never had contact with deviants have strong negative feelings, sometimes stronger than persons in contact with deviants. My experiences with the administrative staffs of mental hospitals suggests that these persons are much more fearful of the patients than the treatment staff.

Psychodynamic theory suggests that there are mechanisms of defense that are utilized by persons unwilling to acknowledge their own emotions and impulses. Persons with strong feelings of anger, for example, may project these feelings onto others. It is not I who am angry, but they. Mental patients may serve as a convenient target for the projection of collectively held, but repressed, emotions of fear, anger, and embarrassment.

Psychodynamic theories of prejudice have been current for some time. These theories are no longer strongly represented in the research that is currently being conducted on prejudice because of, at least in part, the severe criticism directed at one of the major studies of the psychological sources of prejudice, *The Authoritarian Personality* (Adorno *et al.*, 1950). Although most of the criticism of this particular study was well founded, it would now appear that it might have been premature to drop studies of the psychodynamics of prejudice.[2] Such studies together with future studies of the dynamics of stigma, may afford new insights into the sources of labeling and, therefore, knowledge of origins of the societal reaction to deviance. I believe that both historical and psychological investigations are needed to complement the sociological understanding of the societal reaction to deviance.

[2]For a current review which comes to this conclusion, see Glassner (1978).

Conclusions

14

THIS final chapter recapitulates the theory and research that has been discussed and adds two final suggestions: a recommendation concerning interpretation of psychiatric symptoms, which has implications for research on mental illness, and a theoretical formulation in which the investigation of the causes of mental illness is translated into a study of the dynamics of status systems.

The theory of mental illness outlined in the earlier chapters is that the symptoms of mental illness can be considered to be violations of residual social norms, and that the careers of residual deviants can most effectively be considered as dependent on the societal reaction and the processes of role-playing, when role-playing is viewed as part of a social rather than an exclusively individual system. The two studies presented show that psychiatric and legal screening is typically a peremptory process in which the patient's condition is at best only one of a number of factors which decide the outcome, with social contingencies being of great importance.

The theoretical formulation of symptoms as normative violations places great stress on the social context in which symptomtic behavior occurs as do the findings concerning the near-automatic procedures in psychiatric screening. Implied in these considerations is a relationships among symptoms, context, and meaning that may be of great importance in future research.

SYMPTOM, CONTEXT, AND MEANING

The admission study showed that involuntary confinement in mental hospitals, in most jurisdictions, is usually based on the presumption of illness by the officials. How accurate is their presumption? The officials whom we interviewed felt that in virtually every case, the family or other complainants sought hospitalization only after exhausting all other alternatives. According to these officials, complainants seek hospitalization only when driven to it by the repeated, meaningless, and uncontrollable behavior of the prospective patient. Prior studies provide support for the belief that some families bend over backwards to avoid hospitalization. Yarrow and others (1955) have shown that the defining of repeated rule-breaking as a psychiatric problem is avoided for rather long periods of time.

The officials, then, conceived of the families and other complainants as very reluctant to even consider hospitalization except in cases in which its necessity was a foregone conclusion. Except for some of the court clerks, the officials did not seem to consider the possibility that some of the complainants might have taken action too quickly rather than too slowly. Are there families in which there is "something wrong" less with the patient than with the family? In their study of scapegoating in the family, Vogel and Bell (1961) found that parental inadequacies and marital conflict were often projected onto the weakest child in the family, so that he was "induced" into the role of the deviant. Some empirical evidence for such "induced" roles in complaints about alleged mental illness was found in Philadelphia, where prehospitalization investigation showed that in some 25% of the complaints, it was the complainer, rather than the prospective patient, who was obviously suspect (Linden, 1964).

The clearest example of the bias of the family's complaints is provided in the work of Laing and Esterson (1964). They present detailed discussions of persons diagnosed as schizophrenics, showing that what is represented to be psychotic symptoms is usually rebellion against extremely tyrannical and bizarre parents. Findings such as theirs have given rise to the belief among many researchers that it is often the families, rather than the patients, who are really "crazy," and that the symptoms of the patients are only normal reactions to very unusual situations.

The formulations concerning "family pathology," although they lead to a more adequate perspective, probably represent only a partial resolution. In his paper on the social dynamics of paranoia, Lemert (1962) points out that the complainants who initiate action against a nonconformer may be caught up, with the nonconformer, in a spiral of misinformation, incorrect attributions, and, ultimately, in delusions on both sides. According to Lemert's formulation, it is the internal political and social–psychological process of small groups that can lead to extrusion, first informally, and later, formally, from the group. Thus, the determinants of extrusion may lie not in pathology of the complainants but in the social-psychological situation in the host group, which may generate elementary collective behavior.

Lemert's paper also may serve as a corrective to the view that only the family setting can lead to the kind of nonconforming behavior which is labeled as mental illness. The small groups which Lemert discusses are not in families but in organizations: factions in businesses, factories, and schools. Obviously, however, the faction politics, selective perception, and the attenuation and breakdown of communication between the suspect individual and the rest of the group can occur in families in ways similar to those described by Lemert in large organizations.

Like Laing and Esterson, Lemert indicates that psychiatric symptoms can be understood if seen in the context of the family or group situation in which they occurred. The grave weakness of psychiatric decision making is the absence of the situational elements. As one psychiatrist has recently pointed out:

> A major source of difficulty in psychiatric diagnosis and evaluation is that symptoms are considered to be pathological manifestations *regardless of the context in which they appear. In themselves, however, symptoms are neither normal nor abnormal:* they derive significance only in relation to the [situation in which they occur] [Coleman, 1964; emphasis added].

The refraction that occurs because the context is omitted in psychiatric examinations is nicely documented by Laing and Esterson (1964). With symptom after symptom, they are able to point out how meaningful behavior, when taken out of context, is perceived to be a psychiatric symptom.

To take the first case they discuss, Maya, a 28-year-old mental patient, was diagnosed at 18 years of age as a paranoid schizophrenic, with various symptoms such as auditory hallucinations, ideas of reference and influence, and varying delusions of persecution. Through lengthy and detailed interviews with the patient and her parents, Laing and Esterson (1964) were able to put these symptoms in a very different light. By probing into an incident in which the auditory hallucinations were alleged to have occurred, the patient was led to these statements: "She said she had felt quite well at the time: she did not feel that it had to do with her illness. She was responsible for it. She had not been told to act like that by her voices. *The voices, she said, were her own thoughts, anyway* [p. 25; emphasis added]." With regard to the alleged ideas of influence, Laing and Esterson found over a year after they began to interview the family, that the father and mother had the idea that Maya could read their thoughts, and that they (the parents) had actually tested her "powers" with experiments in their home. Similarly, the ideas of reference were understandable in context:

> An idea of reference that she had was that something she could not fathom was going on between her parents, seemingly about her. Indeed there was. When they were interviewed together, her mother and father kept exchanging with each other a constant series of nods, winks, gestures, knowing smiles, so obvious to the observer, that he commented on them after twenty minutes of the first such interview. They continued, however, unabated and denied [p. 24].

It would appear, then, that the patient's ideas of reference and influence and delusions of persecution were merely descriptions of her parents' behavior toward her. Laing and Esterson document many such misinterpretations in all of the cases they studied.[1]

How do such glaring misinterpretations occur in psychiatric screening? One obvious cause is simple lack of information. Lemert worked for several years in collecting information about eight cases from interviews with relatives, neighbors, physicians, employers, police, attorneys, and jury members. Laing and Esterson spent an average of 25 hours in interviewing each of the 11 families in their study, with a range of from 16 to 50 hours per family. It is obvious that the kind of contextual information that they uncovered could not be collected in an ideal psychiatric interview of 1 or 2 hours, much less in the psychiatric interviews we observed in Midwestern State, which took from 5 to 17 minutes.

One reason, then, that the behavior of alleged mental patients is thought to be meaningless is that the extremely brief and peremptory psychiatric and judicial interviews shear away most of the information about the context in which the "symptomatic" behavior occurred. There is another kind of factor which leads to the presumption of illness, however, which is more or less independent of the amount of time taken in screening. The medical model, in which nonconforming behavior tends to be seen as a symptom of "mental illness," leads in itself to the ignoring of context (Goffman, 1961). The concept of *disease,* as it is commonly understood, refers to a process which occurs within the body of an individual. Psychiatric symptoms, therefore, are conceived to be a part of a system of behavior which is located entirely within the patient and which is independent of the social context within which the "symptoms" occur.

It is almost a truism, however, among social psychologists and students of language that the meaning of behavior is not primarily a property of the behavior itself, but of the relation between the behavior and the context in which it occurs. In his paper, Garfinkel (1964) has shown how even the most routine and conventional behavior loses its meaning when the penumbra of subtle but multitudinous understandings is omitted. The medical model, since it is based on a conception of physical, rather than social events, fractures the figure–ground relationship between behavior and social context, leading almost inevitably to a bias of seeing suspect behavior as meaningless. Given such a bias, even very extensive and detailed psychiatric interviews would not guarantee against a presumption of illness.

This discussion suggests that both the theory and practice of psychiatric screening tends to be biased toward seeing behavior of the alleged mentally ill as meaningless and, therefore, as symptomatic. The practice of screening, by its brevity, tends to omit contextual information, and the theory, based as it is on the medical model, tends to ignore the contextual information that is available. The remainder of this section is devoted to a brief discussion of some of the im-

---

[1] It should be noted that neither Lemert nor Laing and Esterson *demonstrates* their hypotheses, since their techniques are not rigorously systematic. Their findings and similar findings by others, however, appear to constitute sufficiently weighty evidence to suggest the need for research that departs radically from conventional psychiatric assumptions.

plications of these findings for theory and method in the field of abnormal psychology.

Perhaps the clearest implication is the gross unreliability of psychiatric diagnosis as an indication of anything about the behavior of the mental patient. The process of psychiatric screening would appear to be more sensitive to economic, political, and social–psychological pressures on the screening agents than to most aspects of the patient's behavior. This proposition suggests that a basic reorientation is needed in psychological theory and research concerning "mental illness." Too often psychologists and other social scientists simply accept the results of the psychiatric screening process as essentially valid. It is a great convenience to the researcher, after all, to accept society's ready-made measurement of that difficult and elusive dependent variable, psychiatric abnormality, so that he is free to make precise, reliable, and valid measurements of his favorite independent variables. Because of this acceptance, there is now an alarmingly large number of studies which present the ludicrous situation in which there is a refined and sophisticated handling of the independent variable, whether it be genetic, biochemical, psychological, cultural, or a host of others; the measurement of "mental illness," however, is left to the obscure, almost unknown, vagaries of the process of psychiatric screening.

The acceptance of society's official diagnosis is also convenient for the researcher, because it aligns him with the status quo, thus avoiding almost certain conflict with the agencies (such as the hospitals and courts) whose cooperation he needs in order to carry out his research. For the psychologist, it is particularly tempting to accept the societal diagnosis, because most of the common psychological concepts refer to endopsychic processes. Like society, the psychologist may find it much more convenient to locate his concerns in the captive persons of the patients than in the less easily controlled and investigated processes that occur in the wold outside.

To put research into "mental illness" on a scientific basis and to avoid the situation in which the researcher himself becomes one more arm of the societal reaction to nonconformity, it would seem that the medical model and its attendant psychiatric classifications would need to be eliminated from the program of research. Three areas particularly seem to require such reorientation. Those psychologists who seek the causes of nonconforming behavior should measure their dependent variable behaviorally and independently of the official societal reaction. Although there have been studies of "mental illness" in which the research has conceptually and operationally defined the dependent variable, the usual pattern is for the study to depend directly or indirectly (as in "known-group" validation) on the societal diagnosis.

A second research area is in the investigation of the micropolitical and social–psychological process of extrusion in small groups such as families, organizational factions, and neighborhood groups. Very little systematic information is now available on the conditions under which extrusion occurs and on the functions which it fulfills for the group.

A third and final areas suggested by this discussion for systematic research is on the dynamics of decision making in welfare and control agencies. The processes of information transmission, selective perception, and agency–client conflict in these agencies have received little attention from scientific investigators. One example of the type of study needed is an investigation of epidemiological differences in rates of mental illness in terms less of the incidence of disease than in variations in administrative process. A second example of organizational research would concern decision making in treatment processes. A description of this type follows.

TYPIFICATION IN DIAGNOSIS

In the following discussion, I wish to indicate one particular avenue of research that would move outside of the traditional research perspective in rehabilitation. The subject of this discussion is diagnostic, prognostic, and treatment stereotypes of officials and clients and the ways in which these influence treatment processes. Following Sudnow, I use the generic term, *normal cases.* The discussion begins with a review of Balint's concepts concerning doctor–patient relationships.

One of Balint's conclusions is that there is an apostolic function, that is, that doctors in some ways function as apostles, seeking to proselytize their patients into having the kinds of diseases that the doctor thinks are conceivable in their cases (p. 216). It would be easy to accept Balint's statement concerning apostolic mission as academic hyperbole, which is used to make a subtle point concerning physical and psychiatric diagnosis. However, one can also take Balint's statement as literally true and talk about the kinds of organizations and the kinds of situations in which diagnostic stereotypes are used in classifying clientele and become the base for action.

The literal use of such stereotypes is apparent in Sudnow's ''Normal Crimes'' (1965). Making observations in the public defender's office in the court of a large city, he notes that the effective diagnostic unit for the public defender is the *typical* kind of crime: that is, crime typical for this city (the city that he describes) and this time in history. He describes burglary, child molestation, assault with a deadly weapon, and other crimes in terms of the folklore about these crimes that exists in the court in that particular city. To say that this is folklore is not to say that it is completely or even mostly inaccurate. The point that is made, however, is that the thinking of the public defender is in terms of these stereotypic crimes, and his questioning of the defendant is not so much an attempt to find the particular dimensions and aspects of the situation in which the defendant finds himself but almost entirely the extent to which this defendant seems to fit into the stereotyped category of criminal that exists in the court.

I will not attempt to repeat details of this article here. The point that is relevant is that these stereotypes are the functional units which are used by the public defender and, apparently, to a large extent, by the public prosecutor also in carrying out the business of the court. In this particular case, also, it should be noted that the aim of the public defender in using these stereotypes is not so much an attempt to get an acquittal but a reduction of sentence. This technique is, therefore, a way of maintaining a smooth-running operation of the court without gross violation of either the court's concept of punishment, on the one hand, or the defendant's rights, on the other.

It seems likely that such diagnostic stereotypes function in many kinds of treatment, control, and welfare agencies. As the functional units in which business gets done, it is important to note, however, that these diagnostic packages are of different importance in different kinds of organizations and situations. In the kind of situation which one may find, say, in the surgical ward of an outstanding hospital, one would assume that diagnostic stereotypes are used as preliminary hypotheses, which are retained or rejected on the basis of further investigation—that is, at one pole of the organizational continuum. At the other pole, in the kind of situation which Sudnow describes, these stereotyped are not only first hypotheses but also the final result of the investigation. That is, there is a tendency to accept these stereotyped descriptions with a very minimal attempt to see if they fit the particular case at hand. Later in this discussion, I state some propositions which relate the type of situation, the type of organization, and the functional importance of the diagnostic stereotypes.

The idea of "normal cases" would seem to offer an entering wedge for research in the most diverse kinds of agencies. In current medical practice, the dominant perspective is the "doctrine of specific etiology" (Dubois, 1961). This perspective, largely an outgrowth of the successful application of the germ theory of disease, gives rise to the stance of "scientific medicine" in which the conceptual model of disease is a determinate system. The four basic components of this system are a single cause (usually a pathogen in the body), a basic lesion, uniform and invariant symptoms, and regularly recurring outcome, usually damage to the body or death if medical intervention is not forthcoming.

The model of disease in scientific medicine gives rise to "normal cases" in which diagnosis, prognosis, and treatment are somewhat standardized. (Thus, diabetes melitus is a disease in which the basic lesion is glucose intolerance, primary features are nutritional and metabolic disorders and susceptibility to infection, secondary features are retinopathy, coronary heart disease, renal disease, or neuropathy, and treatment is by routine insulin control.) An important component of this disease model is the application for treatment by the patient with complaints which are traceable to the disease. (Feinstein [1963] uses the term *lanthanic* for patients who have the disease but either do not have complaints or whose complaints do not result in application for treatment.) Cases in which the disease is present but the symptoms are not are obvious deviations from the "normal case" and cause difficulties in medical practice and research. Equally troublesome are causes in which the primary or secondary features of the disease are present but in which the basic lesion is absent. Meador (1965) has suggested, only half in jest, that such conditions be given specific medical status as "nondiseases."

The concept of *normal cases* is closely connected with the notion, in medicine, that physicians have of "What's going around." That is, in a normal practice, a physician is not exposed to all kinds of the most diverse diseases that are described in medical textbooks but only rather a small sample of diseases which come in repeatedly: colds, flu, appendicitis, nervous headaches, low back pain, etc.

Proportionately as the case load increases, or inversely as the amount of time that the physician has for each case, as the amount of time that the physician has for each case, as the amount of interest he has, or the amount of knowledge he has "increases," one would expect that these diagnostic stereotypes would play an important role. Some of the atrocity tales of medical practice in armed services or in industry suggest the kinds of eventualities that can occur. For example, at the extreme, in some medical clinics for trainees in the army, virtually all treatments fall into one or two categories—aspirins for headaches and antihistamines for colds, and possibly a third category—a talk with a commanding officer for the residual category of malingerers.[2]

It is conceivable that the same kinds of conceptual packages would be used in other kinds of treatment, welfare, and control agencies. Surely in rehabilitation agencies, the conceptual units which the working staff uses cover only a rather limited number of contingencies of disability, placement possibilities, and client attitudes. The same minimal working concepts should be evident in such diverse areas as probation and parole, divorce cases, adoption cases, police handling of juveniles, and in the area of mental health.

Perhaps the most important characteristic of normal diagnoses, prognoses, and treatments is their validity. How accurate are the stereotypes that agency workers and patients use in considering their situations? One would guess that validity of stereotypes is related to their precision. Other things being equal, the more precise the stereotypes, the more ramified they are in the various characteristics of the client, the situation, and the community, the more accurate one would guess that they would be. Proposition 1, therefore, concerns simply the number of the different stereotypes that are used in an agency. One would guess that validity and precision are correlated. That is, the more numerous the stereotypes that are actually used in the agency, the more precise they will be, and the more precise they will be, the more valid they will be.

Proposition 2 concerns the power of clients. Using the term *marginality* in the sense used by Krause, the more marginal the patients, the less numerous, precise, and valid the stereotypes will be (1900; cited by Myers, 1965). That is, the more the status of the client is inferior to and different from that of the staff, whether because of economic position, ethnicity, race, education, etc., the more inaccurate and final the normal cases will be.

Proposition 3 concerns: The less dependent the agent is upon the client's good will, the less precise and valid the stereotypes will be. In the situation of private

[2]*Cf.* Roth (1962:46-56).

practice, where the physician is dependent for remuneration upon the patient, one is more likely to find a situation at outlined by Balint (1957: 18), where decision concerning the patient's diagnosis becomes a matter of bargaining. This discussion qualifies Balint's formulation by suggesting that bargaining or negotiation is a characteristic of a medical service in which patients are powerful, such that the diagnostic stereotypes of the physician are confronted by the diagnostic stereotypes of the patient, and that the patient has some power to regulate the final diagnosis.

Proposition 4 relates to the body of knowledge in the agency or profession which is handling the clients. One would suspect that the more substantial or scientific the body of knowledge, the less important, the more valid, and the more accurate the conceptual packages. In areas of general medicine, for example, such as pneumonia and syphilis, the kind of stereotyping process discussed here is relatively unimportant. The same would be true in some areas of physical rehabilitation.

Proposition 5 relates the socialization of the staff member to his use of conceptual packages. One would assume that a fairly accurate index of socialization into an agency would be the degree to which a staff member uses the diagnostic packages that are prevalent in that agency. This proposition suggests a final proposition that is somewhat more complicated, relating effectiveness of a staff member in diagnosis or prognosis to his use of diagnostic stereotypes. One would guess that effectiveness has a curvilinear relationship to knowledge and use of stereotypes. In the beginning, a new staff member would have only theory and little experience to guide him and would find that his handling of clients is time-consuming and his diagnoses tend to be inaccurate. As he learns the conceptual packages, he becomes more proficient and more rapid in his work, so that effectiveness increases. The crucial point comes after a point in time in which he has mastered the diagnostic packages, and the question becomes, is his perceptiveness of client situations and placement opportunities going to remain at this stereotypic level, where it is certainly more effective than it was when he was a novice in the organization? Is it going to become frozen at this stereotypic level or is he going to go on to begin to use these stereotypes as hypotheses for guiding further investigation on his part? I would suggest that this is a crucial point in the career of any staff member in an agency, and the research which would tell us about this crisis would be most beneficial.[3]

Although carrying out research with normal cases could involve fairly complex procedures (i.e., in checking on the validity of diagnostic stereotypes in a series of cases), the beginning efforts in research could be fairly simple. One of the first questions I would want to ask in beginning a study of this kind would be something like, "What kinds of cases do you see most of here in this agency?"

---

[3]C. Spaulding has suggested the proposition that typification practices in organizations are also a function of hierarchical position: The higher a person is in the hierarchy (and therefore the more removed from organizational routine), the less stereotyped are his typifications.

With only a little elaboration, I believe such a question would elicit some of the standard stereotypes from most agency staff. Just describing the structure of the normal cases in an agency would be a major step in understanding how that organization functions.

A more ambitious program of research into diagnostic and prognostic treatment stereotypes would be to relate them in each case with the actual outcome of the case. An intermediate stage of research would be represented by any type of gaming study in which experienced, knowledgeable professionals would be assigned simulated cases given information which was found to be the prototypic information used in a given agency. A device for this purpose has been developed by Leslie Wilkins, as found in the appendix of his book on social deviance (1965: 294-304). Wilkins calls this device an "information board." It contains a large number of items, say 50 items, in which the classification of information from a case history appears on separable index cards with titles of the information appearing on the visible edge of the cards. For example, in the work with probation officers that he did as a pilot study, the information board contained charge, complainant's account of incident, co-defendant's account of incident, offender's account of incident, general appearance of the offender, sex and age of the offender, scholastic attainment, practical handling of problems by the offender, attitudes toward authority, and so on. In the various games that Wilkins had these probation trainees play, he allowed them to select several items from the possible list and then make a decision. With a little experimentation, it should not be difficult to devise diagnostic games with an information board which could be played by the staff of almost any kind of agency.

The two principal kinds of information needed in the proposed research would be, first, of the kind of dimensions of client condition or behavior that the staff actually uses in its day-to-day decision making, whether these be blood pressure, race, continence, attitude toward authority, activity level, prior history of sexual propriety, and so on and, second, the constellations of values of these dimensions into which the staff (and clients) combine these elements of information into "normal cases."

Conceptually, there remain a number of difficulties. In some ways, this kind of research is congenial to the approach anthropologists take toward the medical institutions of a small society: the approach to "folk medicine." Anthropological studies of folk medicine seek to describe the medical institutions of a society without accepting the underlying presuppositions of that society. In the same way, the approach to rehabilitation process by way of normal cases seeks to study the flow of business in an organization without accepting the presuppositions of the staff and clients involved. It should be remembered in this connection, however, that in many organizations, there are at least two sets of folk involved, staff and clients, each possibly having vastly different sets of folk categories of illness or guilt, etc.

From the point of view of orderly conceptual formulation, none of the concepts used in this discussion (e.g., *diagnostic stereotypes, normal cases,* and *conceptual packages*) is particularly satisfactory. The concept of *stereotypes* implies more distortion than is intended and does not articulate very well with organizational structure.[4] *Normal cases* is a good enough general term but does not lead to a more detailed breakdown of sub-elements.[5] *Conceptual packages* is much too general a term. Perhaps the best set of concepts would be taken from role analysis. Normal cases imply a set of role expectations which articulate with the position of the perceiver in the organization. Diagnostic stereotypes in medicine, for example, may be construed as the counterrole variants that make up the physicians' role-set for patients. The concept of *role* seems somewhat static for this use and does not immediately suggest conceptual analogies for prognostic (role-futures?) or treatment stereotypes. Perhaps some of these difficulties can be removed through further discussion.

One way of conceptualizing the problem in a broader context is in terms of the *work system* in organizations. Often there is considerable difference between the official version of the work done in an organization and what actually gets done. The preceding discussion suggests that there may be a relatively small number of dimensions which determine the actual work system: the typifications previously described, the consensus on work rates (suggested by Howard Becker), and the precision and dependability with which work output is measured, for example. These dimensions provide the bare suggestions that the culture of the workplace may be considered to be an overdetermined, self-maintaining system and should, therefore, be studied as an analytical whole.

The purpose of these comments has been to formulate the kind of research which would avoid the undue emphasis on the individual and the physical as well as other presuppositions of the professionals who specialize in the rehabilitation process. This difference of viewpoint from those used in the agencies would likely cause some practical difficulties in carrying out research of this kind. Difficulties of a methodological and conceptual character have already been alluded to. Nevertheless, the program of research suggested here may provide a useful approach to a large number of problems in rehabilitation and medical organizations.

MENTAL ILLNESS AND SOCIAL STATUS

It would appear that the looseness of psychiatric theory and procedures, interacting with the attitudes of persons in the community, welfare, and control agencies gives rise to a situation in which individualistic concepts, whether medical or psychological, can explain only part of the variation in the handling of the mentally ill. It has been suggested here that the serious student of regularities in our society may find it profitable to study ''mental illness'' in terms of ''career contingencies'' (as in the study of decision making in the release of mental

---

[4]D. Zimmerman called my attention to Schutz's term, *typifications*.

[5]M. Loeb has suggested to me that ''standard cases'' would be preferable terminology.

patients from mental hospitals in Chapter 6), which govern passage between the status of the ordinary citizen and that of the mental patient.

Sociologically, a status is defined as a set of rights and duties. Although we tend to take the rights and duties of the ordinary citizen for granted, it becomes clear that there is an extensive set of rights and duties which define the status of the sane when we realize the rights which are abridged when a person is declared mentally incompetent (i.e., roughly speaking, when he is committed to a mental hospital). The following is a partial list of such rights:

LEGAL AREAS INVOLVING COMPETENCY

1. Making a will (testamentary capacity)
2. Making a contract deed, sale
3. Being responsible for a criminal act
4. Standing trial for a criminal charge
5. Being punished for a criminal act
6. Being married
7. Being divorced
8. Adopting a child
9. Being a fit parent
10. Suing and being sued
11. Receiving property
12. Holding property
13. Making a gift
14. Having a guardian, committee, or trustees
15. Being committed to a mental institution
16. Being discharged from a mental institution
17. Being paroled or put on probation
18. Being responsible for a tortious civil wrong
19. Being fit for military service
20. Being subject to discharge from the military service
21. Operating a vehicle
22. Giving a valid consent
23. Giving a binding release or waiver
24. Voting
25. Being a witness (testimonial capacity)
26. Being a judge or juror
27. Acting in a professional capacity, as a lawyer, teacher, physician
28. Acting in a public representative capacity, as a governor, legislator
29. Acting in a fiduciary capacity, as trustee, executor
30. Managing or participating in a business, as a director, stockholder
31. Receiving compensation for inability to work as a result of an injury (Mezer and Rheingold, 1962).

It should be understood that this list includes only those rights that are formally abrogated, either during or after hospitalization. Such a collection of abrogated rights points out that there is a distinct and separate status for the mentally ill in our society.

Throughout this chapter, there have been instances in which the mental patient has been compared with other disadvantaged persons of low social status. In this final section, it is argued that it is helpful to make a formal statement in which discussions of mental illness are translated to the language of social role and status; the social institution of insanity can be considered to be constituted by a "status line" between persons designated as sane and those designated to be mentally ill.

Most sociological concepts which have been developed to describe status lines refer to the norms which govern contact between races: the "color line." The structure of a color line, as formulated by Strong (1943) and others is built up around two statuses, the status of the ingroup member and that of the outgroup member.[6] Between these two statuses is the category of exception for persons assigned to neither group. Finally, completing the axis of statuses is the status ideal, which embodies the values of the ingroup, and the negative status ideal, which embodies the vices. That is, the status ideals portray the ingroup hero and villain, respectively. Corresponding to each of the five statuses is the appropriate role, which specifies the characteristics of persons occupying the status (see Figure 14.1).

Applied to the status line that separates deviants and nondeviants, this axis would contain the ideal status or hero of conformity to ingroup values, the conventional conforming role, the categories of exception, which have neither deviant nor nondeviant status, the conventional deviant status, and the negative ideal, or super-villain.

Applied to the status separation between the sane and insane, the negative ideal would be the "raving lunatic" of heroic proportions and other such stereotypes which embody the most intense fears and aversions of the community. The status of the insane would be the conventional negative status, being roughly the status of the committed mental patient. The categories of exception would correspond to such conditions as "nervous breakdown," as used as a euphemism in popular parlance, and "temporary insanity," in which a person's behavior is excused without penalty.

The conventional conforming status would be that of the ordinary citizen whose sanity has not been called in question. What corresponds in our society to the status ideal on this axis of separation? In earlier societies, such a question would have been less difficult to answer, since most societies have held unambiguous and largely uncontested images of the virtuous man. In medieval Japan, for example, the image of the samurai would undoubtedly correspond to the status ideal. In our own earlier history, the members of the "elect," pre-

---

[6]For an application to deviance of concepts drawn from race relations, see Goffman (1957:508).

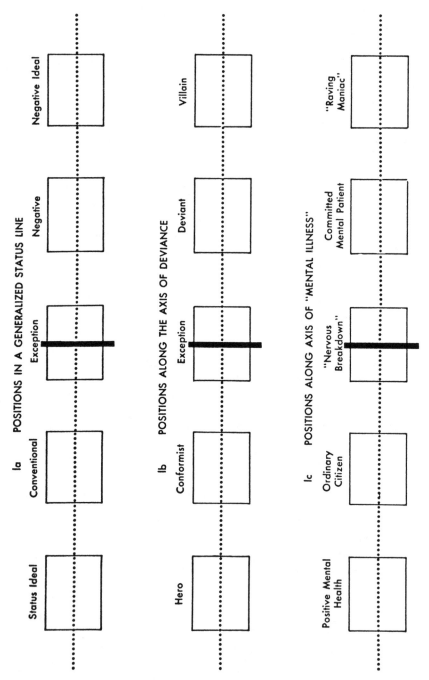

Fig. 14.1. Status lines.

214

destined to God's grace, would also fit this status. In contemporary society, however, religious authority no longer serves to give unquestioned legitimacy to the positive virtues, and the formulation of the role ideal is continuously in process.

It may be that the nearest that our society comes to a status ideal along the sane–insane axis is the concept of *positive mental health*. Jahoda (1958) reports no consensus among psychological experts on the criterion of positive mental health. The following six criteria are among those most prominent:

1. Attitudes toward one's self: self-esteem, correctness of self-conception, etc.
2. Growth, development, or self-actualization
3. Integration of the self
4. Autonomy; independence
5. Adequacy of perception of reality
6. Mastery of the environment

These disparate and conflicting criteria of mental health would appear to be little related to ordinary notions of health but rather formulations of what the various authors regard to be the highest values to which our society ought to aspire in shaping ourselves and our children. As such values, the concept of *positive mental health* comes very close to being what has been described as the status ideal.

Wallace's biocultural model of mental illness bears some resemblance to this model of the status line (1961). Wallace describes five *states* that make up the "theory" of mental illness held by the members of a society: Normalcy (*N*), Upset (*U*), Psychosis (*P*), In Treatment (*T*), and Innovative Personality (*I*). The sequences of states are presented in the following diagram:

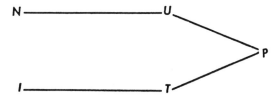

In the case where the Innovative Personality is equivalent to Normalcy, the diagram becomes:

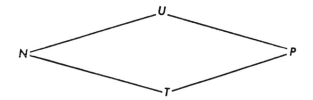

In this version, N corresponds to the conventional status, and P to the deviant status, with U and T representing the unlabeled and labeled phases of primary rule-breaking, respectively. Both of these phases fall on or near the status line that separates the in-group and out-group.

There is one way in which the Wallace model is fundamentally different from the one presented here, however. His model is based on beliefs of members of the society, their "theories" of behavior, and is not directly connected with actual behavior. In the model of the status system discussed here, the positions in the system are actual social positions, each composed of a set of rights and duties, each recognized as legitimate social entities by the members of the society. Corresponding to the transfer mechanisms that Wallace posits (the mechanisms that explain to the satisfaction of the members of the society how the sick person moves from one state to another) would be the actual social procedures in the present model, the *rites de passage* which accomplish the transfer of the person from one status to another. Thus, Wallace's model complements the social system model, since it concerns the individual beliefs which accompany behavior. It would appear that both of the models are necessary to describe the system of behavior involved in the recognition and treatment of mental illness.

One of the most important characteristics of any status system is its permeability, (i.e., the ease or difficulty of passage from one status to another). A status system which is impermeable is called a *caste system*; a status system which is permeable may be called a *class system*. Many of the reform programs that have been carried on in the last several decades in the mass media and more recently in the mental hospitals have been attempts to make the system more permeable, to desegregate first and then, after desegregation, to democratize the status of the mentally ill.

Needless to say, these programs have met with some outstanding successes; it is undoubtedly true that the typical mental patient today has much better chance of passing back into his nondeviant status than he would have 50 or even 25 years ago. It is also true, however, that the status system of insanity still has caste-like aspects, as can be still seen on the back wards of most mental hospitals as well as in many other ways. It is also true that increasing permeability in such a status system means not only that those in the status of the insane can pass more easily into the sane status, but also that those in the sane status can pass more easily into that of the insane. It has been frequently remarked by planners or mental health services that such services appear to be bottomless pits; the more that are provided, the more demand there seems to be.

An interesting, if somewhat unfortunate, consequence of the fact that social attitudes play such a big role in the definition of mental illness is that mental health education may be a two-edged sword. By teaching people to regard certain types of distress or behavioral oddities as illnesses rather than as normal reactions to life's stresses, harmless eccentricities, or moral weaknesses, it may cause alarm and increase the demand for psychotherapy. This may explain the curious fact that the use of psychotherapy tends to keep pace with its availability. The greater the number of treatment facilities and the more widely they are known, the larger the number of persons seeking their help. Psychotherapy is the only form of treatment which, at least to some extent, appears to create the illness it treats. [Frank, 1961:6-7].

Increasing permeability could also mean, as Szasz has suggested, simply that more diverse kinds of problems, welfare, moral, political, are being funnelled into psychiatric channels. In a thoughtful review of what he calls the "inflationary demand" for psychiatric services, Schofield makes the following observation:

It is time for the leaders of the mental health movement to put their minds to . . . analysis of problems which psychiatry and psychology have tended to neglect: to criteria of mental health, to delimitation of the meanings and forms of mental illness, to specification of precisely what are and what are not *psychiatric* problems. It would be a positive contribution for mental health educators to develop ways of communicating to the public on such questions as: "When not to go to the psychiatrist"; or "What to do before you see a psychiatrist"; "What psychotherapy cannot do for you"; "Ten sources of helpful conversations"; "Problems which do not make you a 'Mental Case'" [1964:147].

Both Frank and Schofield seem to be counseling the need for normalization in the face of the tendencies toward routine labeling in the ideology of the mental health movement.

These considerations pose policy problems, which, as such, are not the main focus of this discussion. We have sought in this book to provide a framework which would allow for a disciplined description of the way in which persons deemed mentally ill are handled in our society. It is not intended that this framework be accepted as a precise description of the social system which is operative in mental illness processes but only as a step toward more adequate theory and research. Such a framework may prove useful not only in research on mental illness but also in related areas of deviant behavior, such as crime and mental retardation. As has been mentioned before, race relations also would seem to have structures and dynamics similar to those outlined here.

One field, finally, that deserves mention in this connection is international relations. Perry, in his formulation of "the role of the national," has begun the kind of conceptualization of the status dynamics between nations that has been discussed here for mental illness (1957). Such formulations are badly needed in many areas of social science, since they promise to provide a bridge between social and individual processes. The integration of these two areas of research remains one of the principle tasks of social science. The theory presented here is intended as a step toward such integration.

FINAL COMMENT

This book outlines an approach to the study of mental illness which takes the motive forces out of the individual patient and puts them into the system constituted by the patient, other persons reacting to him, and the official agencies of control and treatment in the society. The theory and the evidence relevant to the truth or falsity of the theory are presented in the first part of the book. Acknowledging that the evidence is far from complete, both in amount and quality, the author concludes that the existing state of evidence favors this sociological theory, perhaps only slightly, relative to the alternative traditional theory based on the individual system model. Obviously, the author is predisposed to accept the theory and may not have been sufficiently impartial in his selection and evaluation of the evidence. Other investigators, more objective than the author, may review the state of evidence and come to a contrary conclusion. Perhaps it may be worthwhile if such a review were made, independently, assessing the state of evidence with respect to each of the propositions in Part 1.

The same point may be made with respect to Part II, the studies of decision making in general medicine and psychiatry. Studies similar to these may be repeated in different settings by independent investigators to assess the validity and generality of the results reported here. Both the review of the state of evidence and the field studies repeating those reported here would likely be contributions to the developing sociology of mental illness.

A more valuable contribution may be made, however, if instead of seeking to repeat the assessment of the literature or the field studies reported here, other researchers sought to modify and refine the theory and research techniques discussed in this volume. The propositions in Part 1, at their best, are very crude statements, lacking specificity and rigor. As Buckley notes in his methodological note (in the Appendix), the nine propositions discussed represent a somewhat arbitrary selection from a larger number of propositions implicit in the theory. This theory, it would seem, should serve as a starting point for the development of a more complete and coherent set of propositions. This set, in turn, could lead to better research and further our understanding both of mental illness and of social processes which regulate conformity and deviance.

In future research informed by this theory, it would be desirable to increase not only the specificity but also the scope of the investigation. A large-scale study which tested many of the propositions simultaneously can easily be envisioned. One such study, for example, would be a longitudinal field study of residual rule-breakers which used an experimental design. In such a study, a survey would be used to locate rule-breakers who have not been labeled in the community. The rule-breakers would be divided into groups according to the amount and degree of their violations, with perhaps one group who repeatedly violates fundamental rules, at one extreme, and at the other, a group of persons who infrequently violates less important rules. Whatever the number and composition of these groups, each would be further divided at random into a labeled group and normalization group. That is, the rule-breakers in the labeled group would be exposed to the normal processes of recognition, definition, and treatment as mentally ill, and the denial group would be shielded from such processes. The effects of the labeling and normalization could then be systematically assessed over a period of time.

To carry out such a study properly, even with a relatively small sample of rule-breakers, would require rather large amounts of money, time, and ingenuity. It would involve some taxing and delicate problems of ethics in research and of the responsibility of the researcher to his subjects and to the community. Nevertheless, if the position discussed here has any validity, if only in small part, the results of such a study could be enormously revealing. The likely conclusion of such a study would not be a clear verification or falsification of this theory but of indications of the conditions under which the social system determines case outcomes: the type of rule-breaker, community, psychiatric or other treatment, and situation in which the social system theory gives a fairly accurate picture of the sequence of events.

Future research aside, how successfully does the present discussion meet its proposed tasks: to formulate a purely sociological theory of chronic mental illness, to compare this theory with current alternative theories, and to judge the relative worth of these competing theories? Some shortcomings are obvious. The exclusion of the personal characteristics of the rule-breaker from the analysis, for example, probably limits the predictive power of the theory. To take just one characteristic: if there is a general trait of suggestibility, as is sometimes argued, this trait would figure prominently in the process of entering or not entering the role of the mentally ill. Contrary to the assumption made here, rule-breakers do vary in their personal characteristics: some have intensely held convictions, some do not; some are sophisticated about legal and medical procedures, and others are not; some are deferential to authority, and so on. These characteristics are probably important in determining how resistant a rule-breaker will be to entering the deviant role when it is offered. Many other dimensions which would qualify and augment the theory could also be pointed out.

As was noted in Chapter 1, however, the purpose of this discussion is not that of final explanation but of a starting point for systematic analysis. To evaluate the usefulness of the theory, the reader must ask two questions: How convincing is the analysis of careers of mental illness, which use gross social processes such as denial and labeling rather than the intricate intrapsychic mechanisms postulated in the medical model? Second, to what extent does the "clash of doctrines," to use Whitehead's (1962) phrase, which is developed here, illuminate the current controversy over policy, theory, and research in the area of mental illness? A definitive answer to these questions may be provided by future research. For the present, the reader must be guided by his own inclination and judgment.

Appendix:
A Methodological Note*

COMPARED to most "theories" in sociology—which are usually more adequately describable as conceptual or categorical frameworks—this theory of stable mental disorder has the rare merit of looking like a theory. Viewed in the stark light of its explicit propositional form, it becomes easy to understand why there are so few of this nature: Not only are they more easily subject to empirical test, but they invite immediate critical comment.

Figure 4.3, a flow chart (see p. 73, Chapter 4) was originally drawn as an aid to visualizing the theory as a whole and the way the various propositions were interrelated with one another. But this led to an interest in (1) the nature and source of the propositions themselves, and (2) the "causal texture," so to speak, of the theory.

For (1), it became clear that in order to complete or bring closure to a reasonable flow diagram of the theory, it was necessary to augment Scheff's specifically labeled propositions or variables with others taken from the textual material. In other words, the labeling of propositions and basic variables was arbitrary relative to other statements and variables in the text equally warranting the status of propositions or formal concepts in a more finished theory. This is indicated in the diagram by assigning numbers above to the original explicit propositions (such as 1, 2, etc.) and adding auxiliary propositions (as 8a, 8b, etc.) that were implicit in the text. This means, among other things, that the reader was forced to build some of the formal theory as he went along, thus, needless to say, introducing another source of arbitrariness and possible misunderstanding.

One lesson here, then, is that each theorist would do well to develop a flow diagram for any theory he may create. For a flow diagram—product of the modern age of computers and cybernetic systems—can be seen as a device of the "new" mathematics and systems research that can represent the logical structure of a system, whether a substantive or a conceptual system. Hence, even in a very simple form, it can be extremely useful in explicating or exposing a loosely verbalized theory.[1] Viewing one's theory in diagramatic form invites the theorist to ask such questions as these: Which statements are to be taken as axiomatically assumed, which are definitions, which are hypotheses, which have a great deal of empirical support, etc. It also makes more obvious, sometimes painfully so, any gaps in the theoretical structure or suggests that the theory remains too indeterminate without further specification of the conditions under which propositions or hypotheses may be expected to hold. And then there is the question whether the presumed theory can be diagramed at all—which may be a question

*By Walter Buckley.
[1] See, for example, March and Simon (1958).

220

of whether the theory has any logical structure (i.e., whether it is a theory after all).

For (2), if a theory is complex, some kind of diagram may be essential to bring out the "causal flow." This is of central importance today as more and more sociological theories take seriously the transactional or *systemic* nature of the phenomena they are attempting to explain.

Methodological orientations used to inform most theories may perhaps be classified into four main types. The traditional causal perspective appeals to one or more prior elements of a complex of factors as leading to the phenomenon being explained. Recent examples are the "funnel of causation" orientation of Campbell *et al.* (1960) and Smelser's (1963) "value-added" approach. Functionalism attempts to work in the opposite direction, seeking to explain a phenomenon in terms of its effects on the complex of which it is a part. Equilibrium system theory, focusing on a mutual interactionism, denies cause and effect distinctions and sees only reciprocal inter-relations. The work of Pareto and early Homans are good examples. But this orientation is of use only for closed systems, having little application to open systems characterized by adaptation, restructuring, elaboration, or evolution. Finally, the modern systems research approach focuses on open systems of organized complexity, which have a history, are morphogenie, and hence continuously elaborate, develop, or degenerate depending on the dynamic structure of interrelations of the parts among themselves and with environmental events. The main concern is to study the various types of complex interrelations of parts or mechanisms that have developed from earlier states and that are elaborating or degenerating in some specifiable ways.

Theories of social deviance can be seen to have run the gamut of these orientations. Earlier simple causal theories (e.g., of the "bad seed" type) have given way to more complex causal theories involving earlier social environment and acquired psychological traits as major antecedent factors. Equilibrium theory sees deviance of elements, such that, after Homans, any departure from the existing degree of conformity to (or deviance from) the group norms is automatically counteracted by equilibrial forces to restore that degree—that is, if the system is a closed one in equilibrium. Functionalism has always had a bit of trouble over the problem of deviance: since deviance is usually seen as extrasystemic and primarily dysfunctional, its universality of persistence cannot very well be explained in terms of the usual functional attributions. Most usually the functionalist shifts gears to an equilibrium and appeals to automatic "mechanisms of control" to handle the disturbing deviance.

As I see it, the theory of deviance that is emerging today—of which Scheff's work is a contribution—is in the spirit of the modern systems approach. This theory see deviance as a system product, one generated out of a complex network of events involving: the historically generated institutional and cultural structure with its vested interests and "moral entrepreneurs"; the matrix of interpersonal transactions within this structure whereby the strains of everyday role-playing generate adjustments, bargainings, and random or trial deviations which, in a context of "societal reactions," may lead to a "labeling" of the self as deviant; the resultant build-up of career deviants—whether aggregates of the mentally ill, subcultures of the alienated, or formal organizations of criminals; and the reactions of these groups directly and indirectly back onto the institutional structure to contribute to its continual elaboration or disintegration. It would seem that any theory that begins to get at the intricacies involved here will have to make use of some kind of tool like the flow-diagram to keep track of what it is saying and what it implies, to reveal the multiple interconnections and the positive and negative feedbacks so necessary to an understanding of process, or structural dynamics, in complex open systems. Thus, the flow diagram in this volume (Figure 4.3, Chapter 4), though only illustrative, suggests some of the intricacies, including possible feedback loops, implied or invited by that theory.

Finally, as theories come to take account of the systemic nature of social phenomena, methodologists concerned with logical implications and empirical tests will have to upgrade their canons of acceptance. It is no longer enough to focus on pairs or trios of interrelated variables and test for correlations. For a theory may be wrong, even though the separate propositions check out, because the variables are not interrelated into the correct overall structure.

Bibliography

Adorno, T., *et al.*
1950   *The Authoritarian Personality*. New York: Harper and Row.
Allan, R. E.
1975   "Medication in the treatment of chronic patients." In Werner Mendel (ed.), *Supportive Care: Theory and Technique:* Los Angeles: Mara.
Aminoff, J. J., J. Marshall, and E. Smith
1974   "Cognitive function in patients on lithium therapy." *British Journal of Psychiatry* 125 (July): 109–110.
Apter, N. S.
1960   "Our growing restlessness with problems of chronic schizophrenia." In L. Appleby *et al.* (eds.), *Chronic Schizophrenia*. New York: The Free Press.
Arieti, Silvano
1955   *Interpretation of Schizophrenia*. New York: Robert Brunner.
Arieti, Silvano and J. M. Meth
1959   "Rare, unclassifiable, collective and exotic psychotic syndromes." P. 547 in Silvano Arieti (ed.), *American Handbook of Psychiatry*. Vol. 1. New York: Basic Books.
Bakwin, H.
1945   "Pseudocia pediatricia." *New England Journal of Medicine* 232: 691–697.
Baldessarini, R. J., and J. F. Lipinski
1973   "Risks vs. benefits of antipsychotic drugs" *New England Journal of Medicine* 389 (August 23): 427–428.
Balint, M.
1957   *The Doctor, His Patient, and the Illness* New York: International Universities Press.
Balow, B., and M. Blomquist
1965   "Young adults 10–15 years after severe reading disability." *Elementary School Journal* 66: 44–45.
Beck, A. T.
1962   "Reliability of psychiatric diagnoses: 1. A critique of systematic studies." *American Journal of Psychiatry* 119 (September): 210–216.
Becker, Howard S.
1963   *Outsiders*. New York: The Free Press.
Bell, Quentin
1967   *On Human Finery*. New York: Schocken.
Bellak, L.
1948   *Dementia Praecox: The Past Decade's Work and Present Status: A Review and Evaluation*. New York: Grune and Stratton.
Benedict, R.
1946   *Patterns of Culture*. New York: Mentor.
Benjamins, J.
1950   "Changes in performance in relation to influences upon self-conceptualization." *Journal of Abnormal and Social Psychology* 45 (July): 473–480.
Bennett, A. M. H.
1961   "Sensory deprivation in aviation." Pp. 606–607 in P. Soloman *et al.* (eds.), *Sensory Deprivation*. Cambridge, Mass.: Harvard University Press.
Bennett, C. C.
1960   "The drugs and I." Pp. 606–607 in L. Uhr and J. G. Miller (eds.), *Drugs and Behavior*. New York: Wiley.
Berger, Peter L., and Thomas Luckmann
1966   *The Social Construction of Reality: A Treatise in the Sociology of Knowledge*. New York: Doubleday.
Berkowitz, B.
1955   "The juvenile aid bureau of the New York city police." *Nervous Child* 11: 42–48.

Berne, E.
  1964   *Games People Play*. New York: Grove Press.
Blake, R. R., and J. S. Mouton
  1961   "Conformity, resistance and conversion. Pp. 1–2 in I. A. Berg and B. M. Bass (eds.), *Conformity and Deviation*. New York: Harper.
Blau, Z. S.
  1956   "Changes in performance in relation to influences upon self-conceptualization." *Journal of Abnormal and Social Psychology* 45 (July): 473–480.
Blumer, Herbert
  1954   "What is wrong with social theory?" *American Journal of Sociology* 19 (February): 3–10.
Bohr, Ronald H.
  1970   Letter to the Editor, *Journal of Health and Social Behavior* 11 (June): 52.
Bower, E., T. Shellhammer, J. Daily, and M. Bower
  1960   "High School students who later become schizophrenic." Sacramento: State Department of Education.
Brauchi, J. T. and L. J. West
  1961   "Sleep deprivation." *Journal of the American Medical Association* 171: 11.
Bronowski, J.
  1956   *Science and Human Values*. New York: Harper and Row.
  1965   *The Identity of Man*. Garden City, N.Y.: Natural History Press.
Brown, E. L.
  1961   *Newer Dimensions of Patient Care*. Part 1. New York: Russell Sage Foundaton.
Bruyn, Severyn T.
  1966   *The Human Perspective in Sociology*, Englewood Cliffs, N.J.: Prentice-Hall.
Bushard, B. L.
  1957   "The U.S. Army's Mental Hygiene Consultation Service." Pp. 431–443. in *Symposium on Preventive and Social Psychiatry*. Washington, D. C. Walter Reed Army Institute of Research.
Caetano, D. F.
  1974   "Labeling theory and the presumption of illness in diagnosis: An experimental design." *Journal of Health and Social Behavior* 14: 253–260.
Cain, A. C.
  1964   "On the meaning of 'playing crazy' in borderline children." *Psychiatry* 27 (August): 278–289.
Campbell, Angus, *et al.*
  1960   *The American Voter*. New York: Wiley.
Caudill, W., F. C. Redlich, H. R. Gilmore, and E. B. Brody
  1952   "Social structure and interaction process on a psychiatric ward." *American Journal of Orthopsychiatry* 22 (April): 314–334.
Chernoff, H., and L. E. Moses
  1959   *Elementary Decision Theory*. New York: Wiley.
Chomsky, Noam
  1969   *American Power and the New Mandarins*. New York: Pantheon.
Clarizio, H.
  1968   "Stability of deviant behavior through time." *Mental Hygiene* 52 (April): 228–293.
Clausen, J. A., and M. R. Yarrow
  1955   "Paths to the Mental Hospital." *Journal of Social Issues* II (December): 25–32.
Cohen, L. H., and H. Freeman
  1945   "How dangerous to the community are state hospitals patients?" *Connecticut State Medical Journal* 9 (September): 697–700.

Coleman, J. V.
   1964   "Social factors influencing the development and containment of psychiatric symp-
            toms." Paper presented to the First International Congress of Social Psychiatry, London,
            August.
Consumer Reports
   1974   *The Medicine Show*. Mount Vernon, N.Y.: Consumers Union.
Coolidge, J., R. Brodie, and B. Feeney
   1964   *American Journal of Orthopsychiatry* 34: 675.
Crane, G. E.
   1973   "Clinical pharmacology in its 20th year." *Science* 181 (July 13): 124–128.
   1974   "Risks of long term therapy with neuroleptic drugs." Paper presented at the Wenner
            Gren Symposium on Antipsychotic Drugs, Stockholm, September 17–19.
Cumming, E., and J. Cumming
   1957   *Closed Ranks*. Cambridge, Mass.: Harvard University Press.
Darley, W.
   1959   "What is the next step in prevention medicine?" *Association of Teachers Preventive
            Medicine Newsletter*. P. 6.
Davis, Nanette J.
   1972   "Labeling theory in deviance research: A critique and reconsideration," *Sociological
            Quarterly* 13 (Autumn): 447–474.
Dawber, T. R., F. E. Moore, and G. V. Mann
   1957   "Coronary heart disease in the Framingham Study" *American Journal of Public Health*
            47 (April). Part 2: 4–24.
Denzin, Norman K.
   1968   "The self-fulfilling prophecy and patient therapist interaction." Pp. 349–358 in Stephan
            P. Spitzer and Norman K. Denzin (eds.). *The Mental Patient*. New York: McGraw-Hill.
Denzin, Norman K. and Stephan P. Spitzer
   1966   "Paths to the mental hospital and staff predictions of patient role behavior." *Journal of
            Health and Human Behavior* 7 (Winter): 265–271.
Dewey, John
   1927   *The Public and Its Problems*. Denver: Alan Swallow.
Dinitz, S., M. Lefton, S. Angrist, and B. Pasamanick
   1961   "Psychiatric and social attributes as predictors of case outcome in mental hospitaliza-
            tion." *Social Problems* 8 (Spring): 322–328.
Dubois, René
   1959   *Mirage of Health: Utopias, Progress, and Biological Change*. New York: Harper.
Dubos, R.
   1961   *Mirage of Health*. Garden City, N.Y.: Doubleday, Anchor.
Durkheim, Emile
   1963   "Sociology and philosophy." In George Simpson (ed.), *Emile Durkheim*. New York:
            Thomas Y. Crowell.
   1915   *The Elementary Forms of the Religious Life*. Translated by Joseph Ward Swain. New
            York, The Free Press.
Eichorn, R. L., and R. M. Andersen
   1962   "Changes in personal adjustment to perceived and medically established heart disease: A
            panel study." Paper presented to American Sociological Association, Washington, D.C.
Eisenberg, L.
   1956   "The autistic child in adolescence." *American Journal of Psychiatry* 112: 607–612.
   1957   "The course of childhood schizophrenia." *American Medical Association Archives of
            Neurology and Psychiatry* 78: 69–83.
   1973   "Psychiatric intervention." *Scientific American* 229 (September): 116–127.

Ellis, A.
1945   "The sexual psychology of human hermaphrodites." *Psychosomatic Medicine* 7 (March): 108–125.

Engelhardt, D. M., B. Rosen, and N. Freedman
1967   "Phenothiazines in prevention of psychiatric hospitalization." *Archives of General Psychiatry* 16 (January): 98–101.

Erickson, Kai T.
1957   "Patient role and social uncertainty-A dilemma of the mentally ill." *Psychiatry* 20: 263–274.

Eysenck, Hans J.
1959   "Learning theory and behavior therapy." *Journal of Mental Science* 105: 61–75.
1961   *Handbook of Abnormal Psychology.* Part 3. New York: Basic Books.

Farber, L.
1975   "Sane and insane: Constructions and misconstructions." *Journal of Abnormal Psychology* 84: 589–620.

Feigelson, E. B., *et al.*
1978   "The decision to hospitalize." *American Journal of Psychiatry* 135: 354–357.

Feinstein, A. R.
1963   "Boolean algebra and clinical taxonomy." *New England Journal of Medicine* 269 (October): 929–938.

Fenichel, O.
1945   *The Psychoanalytic Theory of Neurosis.* New York: W. W. Norton.

Fenwick, M.
1948   *Vogue's Book of Etiqueite.* New York: Simon and Schuster.

Fogelson, R. D.
1965   "Psychological theories of windigo 'sychosis' and a preliminary application of a models approach." Pp. 74–99 in M.E. Spiro (ed.), *Context and Meaning in Cultural Anthropology.* New York: The Free Press.

Foucault, Michel
1967   *Madness and Civilization.* New York: Mentor.

Frank, Jerome D.
1961   *Persuasion and Healing.* Baltimore: The Johns Hopkins Press.

Freeman, J. E., and O. G. Simmons
1961   "Concensus and coalition in the release of mental patients: A research note." *Human Organization* 20 (Summer): 89–91.

Freidson, E.
1960   "Client control and medical practice." *American Journal of Sociology* 65: (January): 374–382.
1970   *Professional dominance.* New York: Atherton.

Friedman, Neil
1967   *The Social Nature of Psychological Research: The Psychological Experiment as Social Interaction.* New York: Basic Books.

Gainford, John
1956   "How Texas is reforming its mental hospitals." *The Reporter* 15 (November 20): 18–22.

Gardiner-Hill, H.
1958   *Clinical Involvements.* London: Butterworth.

Garfinkel, H.
1956   "Conditions of successful degradation ceremonies." *American Journal of Sociology* 61 (March): 420–424.
1964   "Studies of the routine grounds of everyday activities." *Social Problems* 11 (Winter): 225–250.

Garland, L. H.
1959   "Studies on the accuracy of diagnostic procedures." *American Journal of Roentgenology, Radium Therapy, and Nuclear Medicine* 82: 25–38.

Gibbs, Jack
1972   "Issues in defining deviant behavior." Pp. 39–68 in Robert A. Scott and Jack D. Douglas (eds.), *Theoretical Perspectives on Deviance.* New York: Basic Books.

Gill, Merton, Richard Newman, and Fredrick C. Redlich
1954   *The Initial Interview in Psychiatric Practice.* New York: International Universities Press.

Ginzberg, E.
1959   *The Ineffective Soldier.* New York: Columbia University Press.

Glass, A. J.
1953   "Psychotherapy in the combat zone." In *Symposium on stress.* Washington, D. C.: Army Medical Service Graduate School.

Glassner, B.
1978   *Essential Interactionism.* London: Routledge and Kegan Paul.

Goffman, E.
1957   "Some dimensions of the problem." In Milton Greenblatt, D. J. Levinson, and R. H. Williams (eds.), *The Patient and the Mental Hospital.* Glencoe, Ill.: The Free Press.
1959   *The Presentation of Self in Everyday Life.* Garden City, N. Y.: Doubleday-Anchor.
1961   *Asylums.* New York: Doubleday-Anchor.
1964   *Behavior in Public Place.* New York: The Free Press.

Gordon, E. B.
1974   "Addiction to diazepam (Valium)." *British Medical Journal* 1 (January 14): 112.

Gove, Walter
1970a   "Societal reaction as an explanation of mental illness: An evaluation." *American Sociological Review* 35 (October): 873–884.
1970b   "Who is hospitalized: A critical review of some sociological studies of mental illness." *Journal of Health and Human Behavior* 11 (December): 294–304.
1973   "The stigma of mental hospitalization." *Archives of General Psychiatry* 28 (April): 494–500.
1974   "Individual resources and mental hospitalization: A comparison and evaluation of societal reaction and psychiatric perspectives." *American Sociological Review* 39 (February): 86–100.

Gove, Walter, and T. Fain
1975   "The length of hospitalization." *Social Problems* 22: 407–419.

Gove, Walter, and P. Howell
1974   "Individual resources and hospitalization: A comparison and evaluation of the societal reaction and psychiatric perspective." *American Sociological Review* 39:86–100.

Greenblatt, D. J., and R. L. Shader
1971   "Meprobamate: A study of irrational drug use." *American Journal of Psychiatry* 127 (April): 33–39.

Greenley, James R.
1972   "The psychiatric patient's family and length of hospitalization." *Journal of Health and Social Behavior* 13 (March): 25–37.

Griffin, John Howard
1960   *Black Like Me.* New York: Signet.

Gurin, G., J. Veroff, and S. Feld
1960   *Americans View Their Mental Health.* New York: Basic Books.

Haley, Jay
1959   "Control in psychoanalytic psychotherapy." Pp. 48–65 in *Progress in Psychotherapy.* Vol. 4. New York: Grune and Stratton.
1969   *The Power Tactics of Jesus Christ and Other Essays.* New York: Grossman.

Haney, C. Allen and Robert Michielutte
  1968   "Selective factors operating in the adjudication of incompetency." *Journal of Health and Social Behavior* 9 (September): 233–242.
Haney, C. Allen, Kent S. Miller, and Robert Michielutte
  1969   "The interaction of petitioner and deviant social characteristics in the adjudication of incompetency." *Sociometry* 32 (June): 182–193.
Hartlage, L. C.
  1965   "Effects of chlorpromazine on learning." *Psychological Bulletin* 64 (October): 235–245.
Hastings, D. W.
  1958   "Follow-up results in psychiatric illness." *American Journal of Psychiatry* 114 (June): 1057–1066.
Hayward, M. L., and J. E. Taylor
  1956   "A schizophrenic patient describes the action of intensive psychotherapy." *The Psychiatric Quarterly* 30: 211.
Herbert, C. C.
  1961   "Life-influencing interactions." In A. Simon *et al.* (eds.), *The Physiology of the Emotions*. Springfield, Ill.: Charles C. Thomas.
Heron, W.
  1961   "Cognitive and physiological effects of perceptual isolation." P. 8-17 in P. Solomon *et al.* (eds.), *Sensory Deprivation*. Cambridge, Mass.: Harvard Univesity Press.
Hill, A. B.
  1960   *Controlled Clinical Trials.* Springfield, Ill.: Charles C. Thomas.
Hochschild, Arlie
  1979   "Emotion work, feeling rules, and social structure." *American Journal of Sociology,* 85: 551–75.
Hollingshead, August B., and Frederich C. Redlich
  1958   *Social Class and Mental Illness.* New York: Wiley.
Houghton, Neal D. (ed.)
  1968   *Struggle Against History: U.S. Foreign Policy in an Age of Revolution.* New York: Simon and Schuster.
Ilg, F. L. and L. B. Ames
  1960   *Child Behavior.* New York: Dell.
Imber, S. I. *et al.*
  1955   "Social class and duration of psychotherapy." *Journal of Clinical Psychology* 11: 281–284.
Jackson, D. D.
  1960   "Introduction." P. 4 in *The Etiology of Schizophrenia.* New York: Basic Books.
Jahoda, M.
  1958   *Current Concepts of Positive Mental Health.* New York: Basic Books.
Kadushin, C.
  1962   "Social distance between client and professional." *American Journal of Sociology* 67 (March): 517–531.
Kardiner, A., and H. Spiegal
  1947   *War Stress and Neurotic Illness.* New York: Hoeber.
Karmel, Madeline
  1969   "Total institution and self-mortification." *Journal of Health and Social Behavior* 10 (June): 134–141.
  1970   "The internalization of social roles in institutionalized chronic mental patients." *Journal of Health and Social Behavior* 11 (September): 231–235.
Kasanin, J. and L. Veo
  1932   "A study of the school adjustments of children who later in life become psychotic." *American Journal of Orthopsychiatry* 2: 212–230.

Kellam, S. G. and J. B. Chassan
    1962   "Social context and symptom fluctuation." *Psychiatry* 25 (November): 370–381.
Kinsey, A. C., W. B. Pomeroy, and C. E. Martin
    1948   *Sexual Behavior in the Human Male* Philadelphia and London: W. B. Saunders.
Kitsuse, J. I.
    1962   "Societal reaction to deviant behavior: Problems of theory and method." *Social Problems* 9 (Winter): 247–256.
Klapp, O. E.
    1962   *Heroes, Villains, and Fools.* Englewood Cliffs, N.J.: Prentice-Hall.
Koos, E. L.
    1954   *The Health of Regionville.* New York: Columbia University Press.
Krause, E. A.
    1900   *Factors Related to Length of Mental Hospital Stay.*
Krohn, M. D., and R. L. Akers
    1977   "An alternative view of the labeling versus psychiatric perspectives on societal reaction to mental illness. *Social Forces* 56: 341–361.
Kuhn, T.
    1962   *The Structure of Scientific Revolutions.* Chicago: University of Chicago Press.
Kutner, L.
    1962   "The Illusion of due process in commitment proceedings." *Northwestern University Law Review* 57 (September): 383–399.
Laing, Ronald D.
    1967   *The Politics of Experience,* New York: Ballentine.
Laing, Ronald D., and Aaron Esterson
    1964   *Sanity, Madness and the Family.* London: Tavistock Publications.
Lapouse, R., and M. Monk
    1964   "Behavior deviations in a representative sample of children." *American Journal of Orthopsychiatry* 34: 436–446.
Lazare, A., *et al.*
    1975a   "The customer approach to patienthood: Attending to patient requests in a walk-in clinic. *Archives of General Psychiatry* 32: 553–558.
    1975b   "Patient requests in a walk-in clinic. *Comprehensive Psychiatry* 16: 467–477.
Lebedun, M., and Collins, J. J.
    1976   "Effects of status indicators on psychiatric judgments of psychiatric impairment. *Soc. Soc. Res.* 60: 199–210.
Ledley, R. S., and L. B. Lusted
    1959   "Reasoning foundations of medical diagnosis." *Science* 130: 9-21.
Leighton, D. C. *et al.*
    1963   *The Character of Danger.* New York: Basic Books.
Lemert, E. M.
    1951   *Social Pathology.* New York: McGraw-Hill.
    1962   "Paranoia and the dynamics of exclusion." *Sociometry* 25 (March): 2–20.
Lennard, H., L. J. Epstein, and B. G. Katzung
    1967   "Psychoactive drug action and group interaction process. *Journal of Nervous and Mental Disease* 145 (July): 69–77.
Lennard, H., L. J. Epstein, A. Bernstein, and D. C. Ranson.
    1974   *Mystification and Drug Misuse: Hazards of Using Psychoactive Drugs.* San Francisco: Jossey-Bass.
Levitt, E., H. Beiser, and R. Robertson
    1959   "A followup evaluation of cases treated at a community child guidance clinic." *American Journal of Orthopsychiatry* 29: 337–347.
Lewis, N. D. C.
    1936   *Research in Dementia Praecox.* New York: The National Committee for Mental Hygiene.

Lieberman, S.
1956 "The effect of changes in roles on the attitudes of role occupants." *Human Relations* 9: 385–402.

Linden, M.
1964 "Comment," at the First International Congress of Social Psychiatry, London, August.

Linn, E. L.
1959 "Patients' socioeconomic characteristics and release from a mental hospital." *American Journal of Sociology* 65 (November): 280–286.

Linsky, Arnold S.
1970a "Community homogeneity and exclusion of the mentally ill: Rejection vs. consensus about deviance. *Journal of Health and Social Behavior* 11 (December): 304–311.

1970b "Who shall be excluded: The influence of personal attributes in community reaction to the mentally ill." *Social Psychiatry* 5 (July): 166–171.

1972 Letter. *American Journal of Sociology* 78 (November): 684–686.

Lowenthal, M. F.
1964 *Lives in Distress: Paths of the Elderly to the Psychiatric Ward.* New York: Basic Books.

Macfarlane, J., L. Allen, and M. Hanzik
1954 *A Development Study of the Behavior Problems of Normal Children between Twenty-One Months and Fourteen Years.* Berkeley: University of California Press.

Mann, J. H.
1956 "Experimental evaluations of role playing." *Psychological Bulletin* 53 (May): 227–234.

March, J. G., and H. A. Simon
1958 *Organizations.* New York: Wiley.

Marx, Karl
1906 *Capital.* New York: Modern Library.

Meador, C. K.
1965 "The art and science of nondisease." *New England Journal of Medicine* 272 (January): 92–95.

Mechanic, David
1962 "Some factors in identifying and defining mental illness." *Mental Hygiene* 46 (January): 66–74.

1963 "One-sided analysis versus the eclectic approach." P. 167 in H. J. Leavitt (ed.), *The Social Science of Organizations.* Englewood Cliffs, N.J.: Prentice-Hall.

Meehl, P. E.
1973 *Psychodiagnosis: selected papers.* Minneapolis: University of Minnesota Press.

Mendel, Werner (ed.)
1975 *Supportive Care: Theory and Technique.* Los Angeles: Mara.

Mendel, Werner, and A. Green
1967 *The Therapeutic Management of Psychological Illness.* New York: Basic Books.

Mezer, R. R., and P. D. Rheingold
1962 "Mental capacity and in competency: A psycho–legal problem." *American Journal of Psychiatry* 118: 827–831.

Michael, C., D. Morris, and E. Soroker
1957 "Followup studies of shy withdrawn children: Relative incidence of schizophrenia." *American Journal of Orthopsychiatry* 27: 331–337.

Mick, S.
1974 "The foreign medical graduate" *Scientific American* 232 (February): 14–21.

Middleton, R., and J. Moland
1959 "Humor in Negro and White subcultures: A study of jokes among university students. *American Sociological Review* 24 (February): 61–69.

Miller, D.
1966 "Country Lunacy Commission Hearings: Some observations of commitments to a state mental hospital." *Social Problems* 14: 26–35.

Millon, T.
1975   "Reflections on Rosenhan's 'On being sane in insane places.' " *Journal of Abnormal Psychology* 81: 456–461.

Mills, C. W.
1948   *The New Men of Power*. New York: Harcourt Brace.

Mishler, E. G., and N. E. Waxler
1963   "Decision processes in psychiatric hospitalization; patients referred, accepted, and admitted to a psychiatrc hospital." *American Sociological Review* 28 (Aug.): 576–587.

Morris, D., E. Soroker, and B. Burrus
1954   "Followup studies of shy withdrawn children: Evaluation of late adjustment." *American Journal of Orthopsychiatry* 24: 743–754.

Morris, J. B., and A. T. Beck
1974   "The efficacy of antidepressant drugs." *Archives of General Psychiatry* 30 (May): 667–674.

Moses, R., and J. Shana
1961   "Psychiatric outpatient clinic—analysis of a population sample." *American Medical Association Archives of General Psychiatry* 4: 60–73.

Myers, J. K.
1965   "Consequences and prognoses of disability." Paper presented at the Conference on Sociological Theory. Research and Rehabilitation, Carmel, Calif., March.

Namche, G., M. Waring, and D. Ricks
1964   "Early indicators of outcome in schizophrenia." *Journal of Nervous and Mental Disorders* 139: 232–240.

Neisser, U.
1973   "Reversibility of psychiatric diagnoses." *Science* 180: 1116–1117.

Newman, Donald J.
1966   *Conviction: The Determination of Guilt or Innocence Without Trial*. Boston: Little Brown.

Neyman, J.
1950   *First Course in Probability and Statistics*. New York: Holt.

Nunnally, Jr., J. C.
1961   *Popular Conceptions of Mental Health*. New York: Holt, Rinehart and Winston.

Nyswander, M.
1975   "Danger ahead: Valium." *Vogue* 165 (February) 152–153.

O'Connell, R. A.
1974   "Lithium carbonate: Psychiatric indications and medical complications." *New York State Journal of Medicine* 74 (April): 649–653.

Parsons, T.
1950   "Illness and the role of the physician." *American Journal of Orthopsychiatry* 21: 452–460.

Pasamanick, B.
1963   "A survey of mental disease in an urban population: IV, An approach to total prevalence rates." *Archives of General Psychiatry* 5 (August): 151–155.

Perry, S. E.
1957   "Notes on the role of the national." *Conflict Resolution* 1 (December): 346–363.

Phillips, D. L.
1963   "Rejection: A possible consequence of seeking help for mental disorder." *American Sociological Review* 28 (December): 963–973.

Plunkett, R. J., and J. E. Gordon
1960   *Epidemiology and Mental Illness*. New York: Basic Books.

Porterfield, A. L.
1946   *Youth in Trouble*. Fort Worth, Tex.: Lee Potishman Foundation.

Prien, R. F., and E. M. Caffey
1974   "Lithium prophylaxis in recurrent affective illness." *American Journal of Psychiatry* 131 (February): 198–203.

Prien, R. F., and C. J. Klett
1972   "An appraisal of the long-term use of tranquilizing medication with hospitalized chronic schizophrenics: A review of drug discontinuation literature." *Schizophrenia Bulletin* 5 (Spring): 64–73.

Rappaport, M.
1974   "Schizophrenics for whom phenothiazines may be contradicted or unnecessary." Paper presented at the Western Psychological Association, San Francisco, 1973: abstracted in *Psychology Today* (November): 39–138.

Rappeport, J. R. *et al.*
1962   "Evaluation and follow-up of state hospital patients who had sanity hearings." *American Journal of Psychiatry* 118 (June): 1078–1086.

Ratner, H.
1962   "Medicine." *Interviews on the American Character.* Santa Barbara, Calif.: Center for the Study of Democratic Institutions.

Rautaharju, P. M., M. J. Korvonen, and A. Keys
1961   "The frequency of arteriosclerotic and hypertensive heart disease in ostensibly healthy working populations in Finland." *Journal of Chronic Diseases* 13: 426–438.

Report on Texas Hospitals and Institutions
1959   Austin, Tex.: Texas Research League.

Renaud, H., and F. Estes
1961   "Life histories with one hundred normal American males: Pathogenicity of childhood." *American Journal of Orthopsychiatry* 31: 786–802.

Robbins, Lee
1966   *Deviant Children Grown Up.* Baltimore: Williams and Wilkins.

Rogler, L. H., and August B. Hollinshead
1965   *Trapped: Families and Schizophrenia.* New York: Wiley.

Rosenhan, David L.
1973   "On being sane in insane places." *Science* 179 (January): 250–258.

Rosenthal, Robert
1966   *Experimenter Effects in Behavioral Research.* New York: Appleton-Century Crofts.

Rosenzweig, N.
1959   "Sensory deprivation and schizophrenia: Some clinical and theoretical similarities." *American Journal of Psychiatry* 116: 326.

Ross, H. A.
1959   "Commitment of the Mentally Ill: Problems of law and policy." *Michigan Law Review* 57 (May): 945–1018.

Roth, Julius A.
1963   *Timetables: Structuring the Passage of Time in Hospital Treatment and Other Careers.* Indianapolis.: Bobbs-Merrill.

Roth, Philip
1962   "Novotny's pain." *The New York* (October 27): 46–56.

Rushing, William A.
1971   "Individual resources, societal reaction, and hospital commitment." *American Journal of Sociology* 77 (November): 511–526.
1972   Letter. *American Journal of Sociology* 78 (November): 686–688.

Sachar, Edward J.
1963   "Behavioral science and criminal law." *Scientific American* 209: 39–45.

Sadow, L. and A. Suslick
1961   "Simulation of a previous psychotic state." *A.M.A. Archives of General Psychiatry* 4 (May): 452–458.

Saunders, L.
1954   *Cultural Differences and Medical Care.* New York: Russell Sage Foundation.
Schachter, S., and J. E. Singer
1962   "Cognitive, social and physiological determinants of emotional state." *Psychological Review* 69 (September): 379–399.
Schaffer, L., and J. Myers
1954   "Psychotherapy and social stratification." *Psychiatry* 17: 83–93.
Scheff, Thomas J.
1963   "Legitimate, transitional, and illegitimate mental patients in a midwestern state." *American Journal of Psychiatry* 120 (September): 267–269.
1964   "The societal reaction to deviance: Ascriptive elements in the psychiatric screening of mental patients in a midwestern state." *Social Problems* 11 (Spring): 401–413.
1966   "Hospitalization of the mentally ill in Italy, England and the United States." *Yearbook of the American Philosophical Society.*
1967   "Toward a sociological model of consensus," *American Sociological Review* 32 (February): 32–46.
Scheff, Thomas and David M. Culver
1964   "Social conditions for rationality: How urban and rural courts deal with the mentally ill." *American Behavioral Scientist* 7 (March): 21–24.
Schelling, Thomas C.
1963   *The Strategy of Conflict.* New York: Oxford University Press.
Schofield, W.
1964   *Psychotherapy: The Purchase of Friendship.* Englewood Cliffs, N.J.: Prentice-Hall.
Schofield, W., and L. Balian
1959   "A comparative study of the personal histories of schizophrenic and nonpsychiatric patients." *Journal of Abnormal and Social Psychology* 59: 216–225.
Schultz, Alfred
1962   *The Problem of Social Reality: Collected Papers I.* The Hague: Martinus Nijhoff.
Schwartz, J. and G. L. Baum
1957   "The history of histoplasmosis." *New England Journal of Medicine* 256: 253–258.
Scott, W. A.
1958   "Research definitions of mental health and mental illness." *Psychological Bulletin* 55 (January): 29–45.
Shibutani, T.
1959   *Society and Personality.* Englewood Cliffs, N.J.: Prentice-Hall.
Simmons, O. J., J. A. Davis, and K. Spencer
1956   "Interpersonal strains in release from a mental hospital." *Social Problems* 4 (July): 21–24.
Smelser, Neil J.
1963   *Theory of Collective Behavior.* New York: The Free Press.
Smith, M. B.
1961   "Mental health reconsidered: A special case of the problem of values in psychology." *American Psychologist* 16: 299–306.
Snyder, S., S. P. Banerjee, H. I. Yamamura, and D. Greenburg
1974   "Drugs, neurotransmitters, and schizophrenia." *Science* 184 (June): 1243–1253.
Srole, L. *et al.*
1962   *Mental Health in the Metropolis.* New York: McGraw-Hill.
Stokes, J., and T. R. Dawber
1959   "The 'silent coronary': The frequency and clinical characteristics of unrecognized myocardial infarction in the Framingham Study." *Annals of Internal Medicine* 50: 1359–1369.

Stratton, George M.
 1897a   "Some preliminary experiments on vision without inversion of the retinal image."
          Psychological Review 3: 611–617. (a)
 1897b   "Vision without inversion of the retinal image." *Psychological Review* 4: 463–481.
Strauss, Anselm, *et al.*
 1963   "The hospital and its negotiated order." Pp. 147–169 in Eliot Freidson (ed.), *The
          Hospital in Modern Society.* New York: The Free Press.
Strong, S. M.
 1943   "Social types in a minority group." *American Journal of Sociology* 48 (March): 563–
          573.
Sudnow, D.
 1965   "Normal crimes: Sociological features of the penal code in a public defender's office."
          Social Problems 12 (Winter): 255–276.
Sullivan, P. L., *et al.*
 1958   "Factors in the length of stay and progress in psychotherapy." *Journal of Consulting
          Psychology* 22: 1–9.
Szasz, T. S.
 1960   "The myth of mental illness." *American Psychologist* 15 (February): 113–1180.
 1961   *The Myth of Mental Illness.* New York: Hoeber-Harper.
Temerlin, Maurice K.
 1968   "Suggestion effects in psychiatric diagnosis." *Journal of Nervous and Mental Disease*
          147 (4): 349–353.
The Dilemma of Mental Commitments in California
 1967   Final Report: The Petris Committee of the Legislature of the State of California.
Tobias, L., and M. L. MacDonald
 1974   "Withdrawal of maintenance drugs with long-term hospitalized patients." *Psycholog-
          ical Bulletin* 81 (June): 107–125.
Torrey, E. F., and R. L. Taylor
 1972   "Cheap labor from poor nations." Presented at the American Psychiatric Association.
Trussel, R. E., J. Ehrlich, and M. Morehead
 1962   *The Quantity, Quality and Costs of Medical and Hospital Care Secured by a Sample of
          Teamster Families in the New York Area.* New York: Columbia University School of
          Public Health and Administrative Medicine.
Turner, R. H., and L. M. Killian
 1957   *Collective Behavior.* Englewood Cliffs, N.J.: Prentice-Hall.
Ullman, L. P., and L. Krasner
 1965   *Case Studies in Behavior Modification.* New York: Holt, Rinehart and Winston.
Ullman, L. P., and L. Krasner
 1969   *A Psychological Approach to Abnormal Behavior.* Englewood Cliffs, N.J.: Prentice-
          Hall.
Vogel, E., and N. Bell
 1961   "The emotionally disturbed child as the family scapegoat." Pp. 382–397 in N. W. Bell
          and E. F. Vogel (eds.), *A Modern Introduction to the Family.* London: Routledge and
          Kegan Paul.
Wallace, Anthony F. C.
 1961   "Mental illness, biology and culture." Pp. 255–295 in Francis L. K. Hsu (ed.), *Psycho-
          logical Anthropology.* Homewood, Ill.: The Dorsey Press.
Wallerstein, J. S., and C. J. Wyle
 1947   "Our law-abiding lawbreakers." *Probation* 25: 107–112.
Warner, W. L.
 1958   *A Black Civilization.* New York: Harper.
Warren, J. V., and J. Wolter
 1954   "Symptoms and diseases induced by the physician." *General Practitioner* 9: 77–84.

Webb, Eugene J., Donald T. Campbell, Richard D. Schwartz, and Lee Sechrest
   1966   *Unobtrusive Measures: Nonreactive Research in Social Science.* Chicago: Rand-McNally.
Weber, M.
   1949   *The Methodology of the Social Sciences* New York: The Free Press.
Wenger, D. L. and C. R. Fletcher
   1969   "The effect of legal counsel on admissions to a state mental hospital: a confrontation of professions." *Journal of Health and Social Behavior* 10 (June): 66–72.
Whitehead, Alfred N.
   1962   *Science and the Modern World.* New York: Macmillan.
Wilde, William A.
   1968   "Decision-making in a psychiatric screening agency." *Journal of Health and Social Behavior* 9 (September): 215–221.
Wilkins, Leslie T.
   1965   *Social Deviance: Social Policy, Action and Research.* Englewood Cliffs, N.J.: Prentice-Hall.
Winder, A. E., and M. Hesko
   1956   "The effect of social class on the length and type of psychotherapy in a VA mental hygiene clinic." *Journal of Clinical Psychology* 12: 345–349.
Wyatt V. Aderholt
   1974   U.S. Supreme Court, U.S. Law Week (November 19): 2208–2209.
Wyatt V. Stickney
   1972   U.S. District Court for the Middle District of Alabama F. Supplement 344: 373.
Yap, P. M.
   1951   "Mental diseases peculiar to certain cultures: A survey of comparative psychiatry." *Journal of Mental Science* 97 (April): 313-327.
Yarrow M. R., *et al.*
   1955   "The psychological meaning of mental illness in the family." *Journal of Social Issues* 11 (December): 12–24.

Name Index*

A

Adorno, T., 200, *223*
Akers, R. L., 188, 194–199, *229*
Allan, R. E., 146, 167, *223*
Allen, L., 146, *230*
Ames, L. B., 47, *228*
Aminoff, J. J., 169fn, *223*
Andersen, R. M., 86, *225*
Angrist, S., 71fn, 106fn, *225*
Apter, N. S., 4, *223*
Arieti, S., 3, 52, *223*

B

Bakwin, J., 81, *223*
Baldessini, R. J., 167, *223*
Balian, L., 147, *233*
Balint, M., 47, 65, 83, 84, 130–132, 206, 209, *223*
Balow, B., 148, *223*
Banerjee, S. P., 164, *233*
Baum, G. L., 48, 83, 180, *233*
Beck, A. T., 109fn, 169fn, *223*, *231*
Becker, H. S., 37, 177, 211, *223*
Beiser, H., 148, *229*
Bell, N., 202, *234*
Bell, Q., 18, *223*
Bellak, L., 3, *223*
Bendit, D., 70, 71
Benedict, R., 70, *223*
Benjamins, J., 50, *223*
Bennett, A. M. H., 43, *223*
Bennett, C. C., 41, *223*

Berger, P. L., 128fn, 139fn, *223*
Berkowitz, B., 148, *223*
Berne, E., 9, *224*
Bernstein, A., 164fn
Blake, R. R., 53, *224*
Blau, Z. S., 50, *224*
Blomquist, M., 148, *223*
Blumer, M., 178, *224*
Bohr, R. H., 184, *224*
Bower, E. T., 147, *224*
Bower, M., 147, *224*
Brauchi, J. T., 42, *224*
Brill, H., 58fn
Brodie, R., 148, *225*
Brody, E. B., 148, *224*
Bronowski, J., 177, *224*
Brown, E. L., 93, *224*
Bruyn, S. T., 178, *224*
Buckley, W., 72, 218
Burrus, B., 148, *231*
Bushard, B. L., 104, *224*

C

Caetano, D. F., 196, *224*
Caffey, E. M., 169fn, *232*
Cain, A. C., 54, *224*
Campbell, A., 221, *224*
Campbell, D. T., 142fn, *235*
Caudill, W., 65, *224*
Chassan, J. B., 50fn, *229*
Chernoff, H., 87, *224*

*Italic numbers indicate page where complete reference is given.

237

Subject Index